East Providence Public Library
Weaver Memorial Library

APR 2008

LUPUS

W9-BNS-949

NO LONGER PROPERTY OF
EAST PROVIDENCE PUBLIC LIBRARY

East Providence Public Library
Weaver Memorial Library

LUPUS

A Patient's Guide to Diagnosis, Treatment, and Lifestyle

Ana I. Quintero Del Rio, M.D., M.P.H., F.A.A.P.

HILTON PUBLISHING COMPANY · CHICAGO, ILLINOIS

616.772
Qui

Published by Hilton Publishing Company, Inc.
1630 45th Street, Suite 103, Munster, IN 46321
219–922–4868
www.hiltonpub.com

Copyright © 2007 by Ana I. Quintero Del Rio, M.D.

Notice: The information contained in this book is for informational purpose only and is not intended to be considered as a substitute for the advice of your healthcare professional(s) or changes of any treatment recommended by your healthcare provider. Always consult your healthcare provider before starting any exercise program or diet, before taking any medication, or if you suspect that you may have a healthcare problem. No liability is accepted for any consequences of you following or rejecting any of this information.

All rights reserved. No part of this book may be reproduced or transmitted in any form or by any means electronic or mechanical, including photocopy, recording, or any information storage or retrieval systems, including digital systems, without written permission from the publisher, except by a reviewer who may quote brief passages from the book in a review.

Library of Congress Cataloging-in-Publication Data

Quintero del Rio, Ana I., 1963–
    Lupus : a patient's guide to diagnosis, treatment, and lifestyle / by Ana I.
    Quintero del Rio.
        p. cm
    Includes bibliographical references.
    ISBN 0–9743144–3–9 (pbk.; 6 : alk. paper)
    Systemic lupus erythematosus—Popular works. I. Title.
    RC924.5.L85Q56 2005
    616.7¢—dc22   2005002077

Ing. 4/7/08 16.95
Printed and bound in the United States of America

3 1499 00423 4149

This book is dedicated
in memory of my sister, Glory,
and to all the lupus patients.

CONTENTS

)◆

ACKNOWLEDGEMENTS

}◆

I WOULD LIKE TO THANK all the patients, colleagues, and other healthcare providers who wrote about their experiences while living with lupus or working with lupus patients. I especially want to thank my editors, Dr. Bert Stern and Karla Dougherty, for their guidance and encouragement in writing this book. In addition, I would like to thank Jesus Candelaria for the illustrations throughout the book and Betsy Replolge for her help in reviewing this book and providing lay language.

INTRODUCTION

P ATIENTS DIAGNOSED WITH LUPUS (*systemic lupus erythematosus* or SLE) often are so frightened of the consequences that they think their lives are over. This panic is driven by fear of the unknown and misconceptions about chronic (long-term) diseases. The intent of this book is to alleviate these fears and correct these misconceptions.

This book is just what its title states: a patient's guide. It will help guide you and those supporting you through the process of diagnosis and treatment by providing information that lets you understand the medical terms used by your doctor and treatment recommendations given by your physicians. This patient's guide will also enable you to take control of your disease and your life by explaining how to live with lupus, a chronic disease.

Lupus affects approximately one out of every two thousand people. Although there is no "typical lupus" patient, the disease most frequently affects women of childbearing age; in adults, it affects ten females for each male. However, lupus is not limited to women, and it can be diagnosed at any age. It affects people from all ethnic backgrounds, but there is an increased occurrence in minority groups.

How the disease first shows itself ("presentation" in your doctor's language) and the subsequent course of the disease vary from patient to patient. This may be influenced by genes and environmental factors. Consequently, treatment may vary from patient to patient.

Because this book is primarily a guide for patients, you will be introduced to all the various forms the disease might take and to the lifestyle changes that make living with lupus easier. However, this guide is also intended as a source of information for family members and friends who are supporting the patient and for community leaders and allied health professionals who work with lupus patients.

For people who have been diagnosed with any serious illness or chronic (long-term) condition, a positive attitude will provide the strength and courage needed to be actively involved in treatment options and care. A positive outlook also fosters peace of mind, which will help the patient maintain a sense of control over his or her life. So the core message of this book is quite simple: always believe in yourself, have faith, and follow the guidance and advice of your physicians.

Following are two encouraging and inspiring stories of women that will show you the possibilities of living with lupus.

MARY JO GREEN: A LUPUS SURVIVOR'S STORY

We must not forget that lupus is more than a medical problem— it is a harsh test of the spirit. The beauty of this test is that so many lupus patients pass with flying colors. Here is the story of one of those high-flying spirits:

I am a sixty-nine-year-old female and have had lupus over twenty-five years. Because of this disease, there are times I feel so sick and completely drained of energy that I have to stop and rest for long periods of time to regain my strength. Because by nature I am an active person, coping with this feeling of being so tired I can barely get out of bed is extremely difficult for me. I also suffer from minor skin rashes, which are red and rounded patches. These patches emerge when my skin has been exposed to the sun. These skin rashes can develop on the nose, cheeks, ears, scalp, arms, chest, and shins. Another symptom that I am plagued with is ulcers in the nose and mouth. The nose ulcers cause recurring nosebleeds. The mouth ulcers appear throughout the mouth and burn, especially when I eat certain foods.

I always feel better in warm, dry weather; however, I have to avoid being out in the sun for very long. Years before being diagnosed with lupus, I would feel sick and run a low-grade fever after spending the day at the lake, and did not know why. I now know this is because I had been exposed to too much sunlight, which triggered my lupus symptoms to emerge even then. Along with lupus, my arthritis pain causes me a lot of discomfort. I have also developed high blood pressure in the last few years and have to take medication to keep it under control. In addition, I have Raynaud's disease, which is a condition in which small arteries, usually in the fingers and toes, go into spasm, causing the skin to become pale or patchy red to blue. This causes poor circulation in both the hands and feet.

After menopause, I showed major improvement in my lupus "attacks" which previously were so debilitating that hospitalization was usually required. These attacks came about when my symptoms were so severe I just couldn't find the strength to continue on my own. Some vital organ, usually my kidneys, would just cease to function properly. Once, I was left in such a weakened state that I had to spend time recuperating in the hospital.

Because there is no cure for this disease, it is my belief that my strong faith in God, and my prayers for strength and guidance, have brought me to this day. I am constantly busy trying to fill my life and mind with other interests. Even though it is not always easy to keep going, I cannot and will not give in to this disease. I have many hobbies and activities that include reading, writing, volunteering with senior citizens, volunteering at nursing homes, staying active in my job, and spending time with family. I also try to eliminate, or at least minimize, the stress in my life. The secret to minimizing that stress is waking every day and thanking God for allowing me to experience another day. I try to do something nice each day, even if it is just a compliment, a smile, or a thank-you. I try to live each day as if it were my last day, hoping to make a lasting impression on those I encounter. This is sometimes hard to do, especially when my own pain and discomfort are constantly plaguing me. However, with God, all things are possible! I also have a loving and supportive family, who have been there for me in both the bad times and good. Everyone should thank God for the good times in their lives. Attitude is half the battle. I may not be able to do much good in the world, but I will continue to strive to be a viable presence in the lives that I do come in contact with, and I hope to make a difference.

Nephrologist Dr. Lucas Haragsim's experience with a patient we'll call Gladys shows that despite complications, with prompt and proper medical care, lupus patients can have successful pregnancies.

Gladys was a nineteen-year-old African-American woman who had had a diagnosis of lupus for approximately six months. Her symptoms were limited to her joints, and she did not have any evidence of organ damage so despite occasional mild joint pains, Gladys thought of herself as completely healthy. But as sometimes happens with some patients, Gladys's lupus progressed rather rapidly, and within a short period of time, weeks in fact, she developed kidney disease. Gladys's tests results were not encouraging. She had rapidly progressing glomerular nephritis with crescents, which is the most dramatic development she could have had.

The treatment that Gladys required is effective if it is given very quickly but the side effects are the loss of menstrual periods and frequently infertility. So not only was this nineteen-year-old young woman facing the sudden realization that she was very sick, she was also facing a dilemma: I can try to save my kidneys but I am not going to be able to have babies, or I can try to keep my fertility but I might end up on dialysis. Gladys decided to undergo treatment until she was started on cyclophosphamide and steroids. A few months into the treatment she lost her periods. But thanks to her doctors, the treatments were successful and Gladys's renal function normalized; she never required dialysis and she continued to make regular visits to the clinic. She finished her course of chemotherapy, continued with her long-term medications, and visited the clinic once a month.

Gladys eventually married, and it seemed that aside from an occasional swelling in her right leg, she was getting used to living with her chronic disease. Two years later, Gladys admitted at a clinic visit that she had stopped taking some of her medications and was now worried because she was experiencing swelling in not just her right leg, but in both legs. In addition, she also had complaints of nausea and vomiting, and overall feeling very unusual—a way she had never felt before. The ultrasound tests her doctors ordered for the suspicion of deep venous thrombosis (DVT) were positive and the scans showed lower extremity deep vein thromboses. But upon further questioning, Gladys admitted that her periods had returned and had once again stopped for about two months. The urine test that her quick-thinking doctor ordered showed that Gladys was, despite the odds, pregnant!

All the textbooks of internal medicine state that pregnancy and lupus do not fit together well so her doctors knew they were in for an uphill battle, especially since Gladys already had a history of deep vein thromboses. She required aggressive control of her lupus but she was adamant about continuing with the pregnancy no matter what the risk. After seven more months of heroic effort and medical support from her healthcare team, Gladys successfully gave birth and was able to go home from the hospital with normal renal function and a healthy baby daughter.

PART I

UNDERSTANDING LUPUS AND HOW TO LIVE WITH THE ILLNESS

CHAPTER ONE

)❧

WHAT IS SYSTEMIC
LUPUS ERYTHEMATOSUS?

L UPUS IS A CHRONIC (long-term) autoimmune disease of
unknown origin that causes the body's own cells to attack
each other. Instead of defending against foreign invaders,
as the body's cells are supposed to do, an immune system affected
by lupus forms *antibodies* against its own cells. These attacks can
cause problems in various parts of the body, ranging from the skin
to the internal organs. The reason why the body turns against
itself in this way is still unknown. Diagnosing lupus can be
difficult because symptoms vary widely from one patient to
another. Lupus can be severe in some patients, and mild in others,
who continue to live normal lives with few complications. It is
important to know that lupus is not contagious; it is not an
infection, and it is not cancer.

The name *lupus* itself helps us to understand the history of
the disease. Lupus was first considered to be a skin disease. The
Latin word for "wolf," lupus was used in ancient times to describe
the rash on the cheeks and nose bridge (*malar rash*) present in
lupus patients. The ancients thought the rash came from an
animal bite; it wasn't until 1874 that lupus was found to affect

various organs of the body, thus causing what is called the *systemic* involvement of the disease. "Systemic" means "throughout the body," which, in medical terms, refers to something that affects the entire body or a combination of *systems* (groups of organs that work together), including the skin, blood, central nervous system, lungs, heart, kidneys, joints, membranes, and other components of the body.

While lupus is most frequently found in adolescents, young adults, and women of reproductive years, the disease can be diagnosed at any time in life, although it is rare before the age of five. Before the age of twelve and after sixty, the disease is equally present in men and women. It has been observed that lupus in men can be more severe than in women. The difference may be explained by a delay in diagnosing lupus in men as men are often more reluctant than women to seek medical advice. Lupus affects people of all ethnic groups, but in the United States, it is more aggressive in minority groups—especially African Americans, Hispanics, and Native Americans. In the United States, the incidence (new cases) of lupus ranges from 2.0 to 7.6 cases per 100,000 people per year. The prevalence (all cases of lupus, new and old) has been estimated to be between 12.0 and 50.8 cases per 100,000 people.

Lupus in African-American patients usually takes the form of *discoid* lupus (a type of rash with red, raised patches with scaling of the overlying skin). It can affect the kidneys, muscles, and the heart. In Caucasians and Hispanics, there tend to be more *malar* rashes (the previously mentioned "butterfly-shaped" red rash, which may be flat or raised, over the cheeks below the eyes), photosensitivity (sensitivity to sunlight), and mouth ulcers. In the United States, Hispanics are diagnosed at an earlier age with heart or kidney disease, and in Asians, lupus is especially likely to involve the central nervous system. Across the world, lupus is frequently found in people of Polynesian descent in New Zealand, and also in populations in China, Southeast Asia, among Alaskan Tlingit Indians, Manitoba Algonkian Indians, and in Nuu-Chah-Nulth Indians of British Columbia. Lupus is rare in blacks living in Africa. A combination of genetic and environmental factors are suspected of causing lupus.

There are four types of lupus:

- Neonatal (newborn) lupus
- Discoid lupus
- Drug-induced lupus
- Systemic lupus erythematosus.

This book focuses on systemic lupus erythematosus, but the other types of lupus are described throughout the book as well.

CHAPTER TWO

>❦

LIVING WITH LUPUS

E ACH DAY CAN BE A CHALLENGE for patients living with lupus. While trying to cope with the disease itself, it may become difficult to maintain responsibilities in your personal life and career. Sometimes you may not have the energy to continue your daily routine or even to get out of bed because you feel so poorly. At times like these, you will especially need the support of your healthcare provider and of those close to you. Loved ones can help you through the bad spells, and health professionals can help you, your family members, and others in your support system to understand the disease and cope with difficulties that may arise.

A TEENAGER WHO COULD

My practice is limited to pediatrics, so most of the children with lupus whom I treat are teens. This is a time of great change for children, as they mature into adults. The greatest challenge facing teens is to become independent. When they are ill, however, they want someone to take care of them, and to fix it. When health is threatened, they are most likely to act like a much younger child and try to deny that they are ill. It is as if refusing to admit their health problems could make them disappear. This is absolutely the wrong thing to do with lupus. I particularly remember one boy who developed lupus at age eleven. He had classic symptoms: the rash on his cheeks, continuous fatigue, and arthritis, too. His lab studies showed that he had systemic lupus erythematosus, but it was quite mild so far and no major organ had been affected. I spent a lot of time with him, trying to make sure he knew that close monitoring of any subtle sign of a lupus flare-up would help us prevent damage to his important organs. At first he did well, but then he started to develop kidney problems. He needed several in-office treatments. But after three visits, he stopped coming to the office for checkups .We tried to contact him, but his family had moved out of state.

I sent him a letter that was forwarded by the post office to his new address. He contacted me and said that his lupus was gone—and that it was because he had seen a faith healer. I tried to caution him that without the full treatment regimen, his kidneys would still be in trouble. About three months later, he came back to town, still symptom free, and was out in the hot sun playing with his friends. Of course, since he was sure he was cured (no matter what I'd told him), he was shocked when he developed a rash all over his face, chest, and arms; he also started to feel achy and extremely tired after only a few hours in the sun—with no sunscreen and no hat, of course.

By the time I saw him, everything was back, but worse. His rash was awful, he had mouth sores, his muscles were weak, and his joints were swollen and painful. Worst of all, his blood pressure was dangerously high, and his urine had too much protein and blood. His nephritis (kidney disease) was back with a vengeance. After a stormy week in the hospital, he seemed on the road to recovery. We had a long talk (again) about close follow-up with a doctor to keep the lupus in good control. We discussed how being sick with anything can feel like *he was losing control over his own life—and that it was normal for him to feel that way. We also talked about how it feels to be dependent on medicine, on your parents, and your doctors in a way other kids his age did not need to be. Most importantly, we talked about the dangers of denial and how the best way to take charge of his life again was to take charge of his lupus. To help reinforce his need to be responsible, I challenged him on all his medicines, their names and doses, their dose schedule, and why he was on each one. I handed prescriptions to him, not his mother. I gave him the orders for lab work and put him in charge of calling my office to check up on the results.*

This young man, now fourteen years old, rose to the challenge. He stopped missing appointments. He knew every drug, every dose, and every reason he took them. His kidney disease went into remission, and we were able to stop the blood pressure medicine he was taking completely.

He finished high school and enrolled in a junior college program out of state. He continued to see me during his school breaks (he made his own appointments), and he always arranged to get his lab studies done before each visit. He had a few flares-ups of his disease, of course, but they were mild and quite easy to treat (one was when he forgot to call for refills and ran out for a week before his regularly scheduled appointment).

I am delighted to say that despite very aggressive kidney disease and bad discoid and malar rash, he had no obvious organ damage at the time he first saw his adult rheumatologist at the age of twenty-one. His teenage denial of illness nearly killed him, but it also taught him an important lesson: the key to living with lupus is controlling the disease, and not letting it control you.

Kathleen M. O'Neil, M.D.
Pediatric Rheumatologist

It is my experience as a physician that the more a patient knows about lupus the better able he or she is to cope with it. There are a variety of places where information can be obtained, including books, professional literature, the Internet, support groups, and, of course, from healthcare professionals.

There are many books about lupus, including medical textbooks and books written by patients or healthcare professionals about the experience of living with lupus and suggestions on how to cope with the disease. In the professional literature, you can find a large selection of medical publications covering the different aspects of the disease. Chapter 10 provides a selection of references to these publications, in addition to a wide selection of national and international Web sites concerning lupus and related conditions, as well as the sites of agencies, companies, and support groups that offer services or products. Also, the Lupus Foundation of America's Web site sponsors chat rooms for lupus patients. Most important, Chapter 10 includes a section on how to access medical care and related services.

Joining a support group is a wonderful way to meet other people with your condition and share your experiences. Support groups are usually organized by patients in various communities. Patients who are interested in organizing a support group should contact their physicians, local lupus associations, or the public health department to obtain information and perhaps even support for starting the group. Once the group is formed, it will depend entirely on the organizers to set the meetings and activities for the calendar year. Support groups offer an excellent opportunity for members and the community to learn more about lupus and learn ways to help each other to live better lives despite having a chronic and sometimes debilitating disease.

Let's next discuss some factors and necessary changes in your daily activities that may improve your quality of life while living with the diagnosis of lupus.

DIET

Good nutrition is an important part of the overall treatment plan for lupus. Although there are no specific dietary guidelines for people with lupus, a balanced diet provides the necessary fuel for the body to carry on its normal functions. Patients need a diet suitable to their condition; ultimately, the diet recommended will depend on the symptoms and related disorders that may accompany lupus. For example, a diabetic patient will need a diet for people who have diabetes, a low-salt diet is preferable for people with hypertension or on steroid therapy, and so on. In general, however, baked, steamed, or broiled foods are preferable to fried foods. Some reports suggest the intake of food rich in omega-3 fatty acids may reduce inflammation, but further studies are needed to evaluate if these foods really offer any improvement. A registered dietician can help you design the diet that is best for your condition, take into account any medications you may be taking, and show you ways to stick to your diet. He or she will be able to provide information and, together with a physician or medical team, can help you achieve a healthy diet.

Some lupus patients may experience weight loss or poor appetite. This is frequently seen in people newly diagnosed with lupus who commonly report weight loss over a long period of time prior to being diagnosed. Weight loss and poor appetite can be caused by the illness itself or by medications that cause stomach upset or mouth sores. Weight loss may also be attributed to depression arising from difficulty in dealing with the life changes required by the disease. In your regular follow-up visits, your doctor, nurse, or health team will assess your diet to make sure you are eating properly to avoid further weight loss.

In contrast, another common problem that some lupus patients encounter is weight gain. Weight gain may be a problem for patients being treated with corticosteroids. These drugs often increase a person's appetite, and, if not following a diet, unwanted weight gain will occur. Following a low-salt diet while on corticosteroids will reduce the risk of developing high blood pressure and water retention. The more weight the patient gains without offsetting it with proper diet and exercise, the higher the risk of developing other related disorders.

Your doctor, nurse, or health team may suggest a low-fat diet, exercise, and behavior modification techniques to help prevent unwanted weight gain. A registered dietitian can learn what your favorite and least favorite foods are, evaluate your eating patterns, and then design a diet specifically for your needs and lifestyle. One of the recommendations that the author gives patients is to keep a diary of everything that they eat or drink each day. Recording this information by date and time can help their healthcare team evaluate their eating patterns. This will help identify any behavioral problems of which the patient may be unaware. It is also important to keep a record of one's exercise program, if any. Once patients realize what they are doing wrong, it is easier for them to change their lifestyle habits. This may take several weeks to a few months. It is not easy, but it is not impossible. Remember that you don't need to do this alone; your family, friends, and medical team will help you achieve your goals.

STAYING POSITIVE

For a person with lupus, as for anyone else, having clear and realistic goals and expectations helps you to have a sense of control over your life, to improve your self-image, and to have a positive attitude. You will need the ability to stay positive amidst the ups and downs of the disease interrupting your projects, plans, and obligations.

Family, friends, or an outside support group can help greatly in keeping you emotionally steady and in caring for you when you need help; therefore, it is important to communicate openly with them. Objectively as possible, tell people what you can and cannot do and what you need from them. Help them to understand the disease and the way it affects ordinary life. People who understand are more likely to sympathize and feel motivated to help as they can.

It may take your family a little time to take it all in. Family members may feel overwhelmed at first when they learn about your diagnosis—confused, afraid of the unknown, and helpless. There may be difficult times in which your family will not understand or will ask more of you than you can give them. This is especially true for the families of parents diagnosed with lupus. Initially, your spouse or children may not understand that there will be some days where you feel too poorly to get out of bed. Other times, your spouse or children may expect you keep up with your usual obligations without realizing that you are overwhelmed and physically unable to do everything you used to do before you became ill. Depending on how controlled your disease is, some days you will be able to do everything you have to do, but on others you may be limited. Your family may not fully understand this unless you patiently explain—repeatedly. But with your help, your family, like most, will learn to adjust.

Communication, patience, and remaining positive are the keys for success in dealing with your family and others.

Depending on the severity and fluctuations of your disease as well as your state of mind, you may experience changes in your sexual life. The constant pain and fatigue associated with lupus may make it difficult to cope with the physical and emotional demands of sex. In general, there are several emotional and physical adjustments that might encourage your sexual interest. First, a healthy attitude about life and yourself can play an important part in maintaining your serenity. A positive outlook certainly has a role in maintaining a healthy self-image and positive feelings about your sexuality. Second, a decreased sex drive is a common side effect of some medications. If you notice a change in sexual desire after starting a new medication, tell your doctor or nurse. Third, the pain of the disease may limit your activities, so you can ask your doctor to recommend or prescribe an anti-inflammatory or pain medication. Sometimes it helps simply to relax and ease some of the pain with a warm shower or bath just before engaging in any type of activity, including sex.

Long-term use of immunosuppressive medication may cause vaginal dryness, or even yeast infections, both which can interfere with your sex life. Vaginal dryness may improve with the use of a water-based personal lubricant. Vaginal yeast infections are easily treated, so if you have one, your doctor can prescribe the medication you need. Lupus patients suffering from Raynaud's phenomenon (see Chapter 4) may find that sexual activity triggers its symptoms. This is because, during sex, the flow of blood increases to the genital area and decreases from other areas of the body, including the fingers. The exaggerated decrease in blood flow to the fingers and toes can cause the numbness and pain of Raynaud's phenomenon to occur. To alleviate these conditions, Raynaud's sufferers should increase circulation to their fingers and toes by taking a warm bath. In general, lupus patients should take measures to be well rested prior to and after sexual relations to prevent exhaustion.

Other problems can interfere with sexual activity, such as oral and genital sores and skin rashes. You may feel less attractive because of these conditions that are often difficult to control. Your partner may not understand the changes in your desire, the fact that you may feel unattractive, or the physical problems you are experiencing. He or she may think you are no longer attracted to him or her. If there is some type of physical problem that makes it difficult to engage in sexual activity, it may be beneficial to explore with your partner other ways to achieve mutual pleasure and satisfaction. On the other hand, you may feel that your partner is avoiding you when he or she is actually trying to be sensitive to your needs, or perhaps is afraid of causing you more pain during sexual contact. These issues may be difficult to discuss, but an open, honest discussion with your partner can help you understand the issues affecting your relationship. If the two of you cannot resolve your problems together, seek help from your doctor, nurse, or a counselor experienced in working with people who have lupus.

Lupus doesn't have to mean endless inactivity or an imprisoned mindset. Remember Mary Jo Green's words: "Even though it is not always easy to keep going, I cannot and will not give in to this disease."

By developing new priorities and routines and learning to pace your daily activities, you will experience less fatigue, pain, and injury. Also, with the help of your healthcare team, you will learn how to:

• Recognize the warning signs of a flare-up
• Take your medicines correctly
• Understand their possible side effects
• Communicate with your caretakers.

Knowing that you are coping with your disease in the very best way you can will give you a feeling a control. There is no one "best way to cope." Each of us must learn to endure in our own way, discovering what works and what doesn't, never forgetting that to cope well is to live well.

PHYSICAL ACTIVITY

Although rest is important in managing the fatigue and generalized malaise, too much rest can be harmful to the bones, joints, muscles, and overall fitness: Because lupus can cause fatigue, arthritic pain, and inflammation in muscles and joints, the thought of exercising may feel like a burden. However, it is very important for lupus patients to be active. In the past, it was thought that if you had arthritis, you should not exercise because it would further damage your joints. However, research has shown that exercise is an essential tool in managing arthritis. This section attempts to give you all the information you will need about how to start an exercise regimen and the proper way to incorporate exercise into the management of your disease.

Initiating an exercise program can seem impossible when you have a disease that can be as debilitating as lupus, but starting slowly and making it fun will help inspire you. A flexible and basic program of exercises, including stretching, will improve your range of motion and help you perform your daily activities more easily.

Once you have mastered some basic exercises, you can move on to some easy weight-bearing and endurance exercises, such as cycling. Walking is recommended not only for a cardiovascular workout but also to stretch your joints. If you don't like to walk alone around your neighborhood, you can join one of the many walking groups in your community; some even exercise at shopping malls! If you decide to walk outdoors, remember to look for a safe place to walk. Some patients may prefer to use a treadmill instead, but wherever you walk, it is important to wear the appropriate shoes. You need a shoe that gives you support, such as walking or tennis shoes. In this way you will not suffer leg pain after your walk and you will reduce the risk of a fall. It is also important to wear sun protection (sunblock, hat, long sleeves) if walking outdoors. It is best not to walk between the hottest period of the day (between 10:00 a.m. and 4:00 p.m.) The recommended length of time for a walking program is at least 20–30 minutes each day.

Cycling is recommended for patients with arthritis, especially children, because it exercises all the joints. It is important to ride in a safe place. (Stationary bicycles can be used in the comfort of your home or gym.) When cycling outdoors remember to use protective gear to prevent injuries to the joints or head, apply sunblock to areas exposed to the sun, and wear adequate clothing and appropriate shoes.

Some days pain may make you reluctant to exercise, but remember, the more time you spend inactive the more you are going to hurt. Even a simple activity such as walking around the house can keep your joints moving. If you experience bodily pain regularly, you may want to start with a water exercise program. In the water the stress on your body is reduced, especially on your hips, knees, and spine, making it easier for you to exercise safely.

Water activity, including swimming, is an excellent way for those with lupus to build up strength, ease stiff joints, and relax sore muscles. The water helps support the body while the joints are moved through the full range of motion. The buoyancy of the water places less stress on the hips, knees, and spine. Exercising in the protective environment of a warm-water pool is recommended because cold water can worsen muscle and joint pains. There are some organizations that offer water exercises that are of great benefit for lupus patients and patients with joint problems.

Following a regular exercise routine will help you feel better and you will experience less pain in your joints and muscles. Exercise is also a way to spend time with your family as some forms of exercise such as walking can be performed as a group. Exercising is healthy for everybody—children and adults. Remember, an exercise program can include anything from walking around the block to taking a yoga class to playing a round of golf. Even playing a musical instrument can be a source of exercise, especially if it involves movement of the hand joint. However, it is important to remember not to overdo it, because excessive exercise can endanger your health.

In summary, regular exercise will help you:

- Increase your muscle strength
- Prevent your joints from getting stiff and reduce joint pain
- Keep your weight under control
- Improve your cardiovascular health
- Prevent osteoporosis, diabetes, hypertension, and heart disease
- Reduce stress, decrease depression
- Improve your self-esteem

- Share some fun time with your family
- Help you sleep better.

You should always consult your doctor before starting an exercise program. A physical therapist and an occupational therapist are two other members of your health team who can help you develop a regimen that fits your specific needs and limitations. A physical therapist can show you the proper techniques and precautions to take when performing certain types of exercise. An occupational therapist can show you how to perform daily activities without putting additional stress on your joints and can provide you with splints or assistive devices that can make movement more comfortable. They can also supply you with exercise flowcharts to be followed as a part of your daily routine.

Essentially, a balanced diet, regular physical activity, and a positive state of mind can improve your perspective. Throughout the most difficult moments, there is always a positive way to view your situation. The key is to realize that you are not alone; there is help in the form of family and friends, health professionals, and support groups that can be there for you in good times and bad.

CHRYSTAL'S STORY

Learning to cope with lupus and living a somewhat normal life depends on your attitude and acceptance of your condition. Keeping a positive frame of mind is the key to coping, as are following your doctor's instructions, getting proper rest, taking your medicines as described, and trying to keep from being stressed out. That's what keeps you from having flare-ups and lets you live a prosperous and active life.

}❦

Because the effects of stress and depression can cause physical pain, you need to find healthy ways to channel anger and depression. A strong first step in coping is to work at accepting the things you cannot change, rather than feeling constantly frustrated and upset over situations beyond your control. Hobbies, activities, and regular exercise will help you through difficult times.

You do not have to do all the work alone; it is common for lupus patients to consult psychologists who can teach them coping and stress-management skills. It is also common to see pain specialists, who can evaluate pain, and pain management specialists, who can teach relaxation techniques. The fact is that there are better and worse ways of living with chronic disease. You have every reason to choose the better ways.

PART II

MEDICAL SCIENCES

CHAPTER THREE

٭

HOW IS LUPUS DIAGNOSED?

L upus is a gloriously challenging and horribly unpredictable entity with its myriad number of manifestations and presentations. It can follow the slow steady course of a placid stream for years, easily controlled, even dwindling to a trickle that is barely discernable. In other patients, in different years, it can suddenly erupt like a rain-swollen river crashing over waterfalls, like a dam bursting, out of control, creating untold damage, even loss of life.

We put together all the pieces we have and see if they form a recognizable pattern, one that looks like lupus. Sometimes it takes years to put all of the pieces together for a definitive diagnosis. The frustrating part is when different doctors put the pieces together in slightly different ways; each forms a different picture, and they might not agree on how they see that picture.

Medicine in general is not an exact science and this is particularly true for lupus. One doctor sees a new patient for joint pain, particularly bad in the knees, hands, and shoulders. That doctor notes a red facial rash across the cheeks. He considers a diagnosis of lupus as the potential cause of the patient's symptoms. He orders an ANA, which comes back positive, and treats the patient with steroids. Another doctor sees the *same patient. He just saw another patient with a very similar facial rash, which a dermatologist said was rosacea (a condition unrelated to lupus but which can also cause a facial rash that can be mistaken for lupus). From his exam, he is concerned that the knee and hand arthritis may be osteoarthritis and suspects the shoulder pain is tendonitis. He reviews the lab results and notes that while the ANA is positive, the titer is not very high. He doubts this is lupus at all and recommends stopping the steroids. See how easy it is to be uncertain?*

In this circumstance, without either more experience in distinguishing these features or further testing, we essentially have a deadlock. In some cases even very experienced physicians cannot agree. How to break the deadlock? One way is further testing, like a skin biopsy or joint aspiration or X-ray. Sometimes further testing is not practical or possible and we must then fall back on following the patient over time to see if the picture becomes clearer. If the situation is critical and life-threatening, when we do not have the luxury of sorting it out over time, we may be forced to start empiric therapy even when the diagnosis is uncertain, sometimes even when what we are doing may expose the patient to even greater danger.

All of this uncertainty that surrounds lupus is frustrating for patients and their families. As physicians, we know that. It is frustrating for the doctors too. It is part of what makes it the worst of diseases. We only hope that research into the causes of lupus, its manifestations, and its therapies will someday take away the confusion.

Leslie Staudt, M.D.
Rheumatologist

Doctors diagnose a patient with lupus if the patient shows at least four of the eleven classification criteria for diagnosis as noted by the American College of Rheumatology (see Table 1). These criteria consist of a series of clinical and laboratory findings; there is not a single blood test that can definitively diagnose lupus. The diagnosis is suspected on the basis of a detailed medical history and physical examination, followed by several blood tests. Again, each patient will have a unique set of symptoms and history of how the disease develops. This means that two patients, both diagnosed with lupus, may not share any symptoms at all. Table 1 lists the possible symptoms of lupus.

In lay language, here are the definitions of the eleven medical terms listed in Table 1:

TABLE 1
Diagnostic Criteria for Systemic Lupus Erythematosus

Malar rash
Discoid rash
Photosensitivity
Oral ulcers
Arthritis
Kidney disease (renal involvement)
Serositis (pleurisy, or pericarditis)
Neurologic disease (seizures or psychosis)
Hematologic disorder
Immunologic disorder
Antinuclear antibodies (ANA)

MALAR RASH

A malar rash (or "butterfly rash") is a reddish rash on the cheeks and the nasal bridge (see Figure 1). This rash or *eruption* can be flat or raised, spreading from one cheek across the nasal bridge to the other cheek. Sometimes the forehead is involved, but the *nasolabial* folds (the folds that run from the side of the nose to the corner of the mouth) are spared. The affected areas of the face are those most exposed to the sun (see *Photosensitivity* section). The rash can be present as redness of the skin (*erythema*), blisters (*vesicles*), or bumps (*papules*).

Malar rash is more common in female patients and can be difficult to diagnose in dark-skinned patients. Often the first symptom of the disease, malar rash may appear suddenly and can last from a few days to months at a time.

Lupus patients should avoid direct sun exposure and wear protective clothing and a hat when outdoors. In addition, the

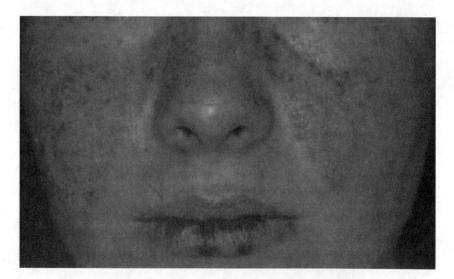

Figure 1. Malar Rash or "Butterfly" Rash

patient should use an adequate sunscreen that contains an ultraviolet-B (UVB) sun protection factor (SPF) above 30. The sunscreen needs to be applied at least thirty minutes before sun exposure and reapplied every two hours during continued exposure, especially when in a sweaty or wet environment. Because water, sand, and even snow reflect ultraviolet light (UV), sunbathing or tanning is not recommended for lupus patients. Ultraviolet light-abating plastic film can be used to cover artificial fluorescent light bulbs and applied to the windows of automobiles and homes.

DISCOID RASH

Discoid rash is a chronic skin condition characterized by raised *lesions* (skin sores) with changes in color or pigmentation, and inflammation around the borders of the lesions. These lesions commonly occur in areas of the skin frequently exposed to the sun, but they can also be present in other areas of the body, such as the scalp, face, arms, legs, chest, or back (see Figure 2) and in the area around hair follicles. Discoid rash lesions appear less suddenly than malar rash, and the duration of active lesions will vary from patient to patient.

When discoid rash lesions first appear, the skin color darkens causing hyperpigmentation. After they heal, subsequent clearance of the center of the lesions may result in scars or discolored patches. Lesions in the scalp cause permanent scarring and may cause hair loss.

Discoid rash is more common in African-American lupus patients than in other racial groups. It is less frequent in children than in adults. Overall, it is present in up to 30 percent of patients with the systemic type of lupus. However, some patients can have the discoid rash without having the systemic type of lupus.

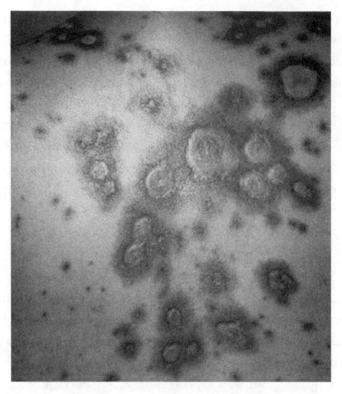

Figure 2. Discoid Rash on the Back of a Lupus Patient

In general, patients with discoid rash need to follow the sun protection measures previously recommended for malar rash. In addition to sun protection, *topical* (applied to the skin) and *systemic* (by mouth) treatments are prescribed. Fluorinated corticosteroids, in cream or ointment preparations, can be applied to the skin to treat the lesions. Gels and sprays can be used for the scalp. In some instances, injections directly in the skin lesions are used when the lesions do not respond to the topical therapy. Special cosmetic products, such as Dermablend® and Covermark®, are available for those patients who develop scarring lesions in the face.

These products not only help the patient's physical appearance but also can act as sunscreens.

Other systemic therapies can be used to treat discoid lupus, such as the anti-malarial medication, Plaquenil®. A patient on the drug Plaquenil® will need careful follow-up with an ophthalmologist because studies show that anti-malarial treatment can cause toxicity or damage to the retina. Additional systemic therapies can be used to treat discoid lupus, depending on the patient's condition.

PHOTOSENSITIVITY

Photosensitivity refers to an abnormal or severe reaction of the skin when exposed to the sun. More than 50 percent of lupus patients are photosensitive. Patient history or physician observation determines if a lupus patient is photosensitive.

Photosensitivity may show itself in several ways:

- An increased sunburn reaction when the skin is exposed to sunlight
- Skin lesions that develop shortly after sun exposure within hours to a few days
- Several other symptoms related to a lupus activation or "flare-up."

Exposure to sunlight or artificial sources of ultraviolet light, such as cool-white fluorescent lamps can trigger skin rash, generalized *malaise* (feeling sick), and fatigue. The sun emits ultraviolet radiation in three bands known as A, B, and C. Ultraviolet A (UVA) and ultraviolet B are directly harmful to lupus sufferers, often causing damage to the skin. Patients with malar rash are more sensitive to the sun than patients with discoid rash. Although the reason why patients are photosensitive is not well understood, it is thought that ultraviolet radiation alters the immune system. The photosensitive reaction may last for a few days. As with malar rash, the best prevention is sun protection—wearing sunblock and adequate clothing.

ORAL ULCERS

Oral ulcers or lesions may be present in the mouth or nose. *Erythematous*, *ulcerative*, and *discoid* lesions are the three types of oral lesions. A patient may have more than one type of lesion at a time. The erythematous lesions are the most frequent. They are usually painless and flat with red borders and appear in the hard palate (the roof of the mouth).

Ulcerative lesions (also known as *erosions*) occur less frequently and may be the result of inflammation of the blood vessels or simply the result of the disease process. The ulcers are usually 1–2 cm in diameter and tend to develop in clusters. They usually occur in the hard palate, but they can also be found in other areas of the mouth or throat. These ulcers may be painful, with a burning sensation or soreness, and may cause problems with swallowing when present in the throat.

Discoid lesions appear as red patches on the skin (*erythema*) surrounded by white dots and may be painful. This type of lesion generally occurs during flare-ups of the disease. Around 16 percent of lupus patients will develop this type of oral lesion. These lesions may become ulcerated, and yeast infections can develop.

Oral lesions occur in up to 57 percent of lupus patients and may even develop before the onset of the disease. They may last for years at a time or in an *episodic* (intermittent) pattern. Usually, they respond to the systemic therapy given during lupus flare-ups. (Refer to Chapter 6 for a detailed explanation of systemic therapy.) Other types of treatments that may be prescribed for oral lesions will depend on whether the patient develops bacterial, viral, or fungal infections. In case of infection, antibiotics and antifungal medication against the specific organism will be required. Gentian violet, an anti-fungal medication, may be prescribed to be applied topically for oral ulcers.

ARTHRITIS

Arthritis, defined as an inflammation of the joint, is one of the most frequent symptoms of lupus. The joints in your body are richly supplied with sensors tied into the nervous system that constantly send information to your brain on joint position, location, speed, and movement. This information is processed by your brain and allows for smooth, coordinated muscular contraction and motion throughout your muscles, tendons, ligaments, and other soft-tissue structures. In chronic inflammatory illnesses, traumas, old injuries, bad posture, occupational, emotional, and repetitive stresses can interfere with this relationship and result in arthritis or other joint problems.

In lupus patients, joint problems may be manifested as:

• Joint swelling
• Morning stiffness
• Pain
• Limited range of motion.

Changes in skin temperature and color may also occur. Swelling, which may last from a few hours to several days or months, is usually *episodic* (intermittent) and often migrates from one joint to the other. In most patients, several joints on both sides of the body may be affected, although the joints of the hands, wrists, and knees are most frequently affected. The spine is less frequently involved in lupus patients than in patients with rheumatoid arthritis. Some lupus patients develop deformity of the joints that, unlike rheumatoid arthritis, does not involve changes in the bone. Joint pain varies for each patient depending on the pattern of involvement, but it is good to note that this arthritic condition generally improves with therapy. Nonsteroidal anti-inflammatory drugs (NSAIDs) are used to reduce inflammation, relieve pain, and help maintain normal joint function. (Refer to Chapter 6 for further details on treatment.)

KIDNEY DISEASE

Kidney disease (renal involvement) is present in at least 50 percent of lupus patients. It is suspected when an analysis of a patient's urine reveals protein or *cellular casts* (a collection of dead cells, fatty granules, or other types of material that form within an area of the kidney). In some cases, a detailed urinalysis that involves collecting all the urine excreted over the course of 24 hours may be performed to evaluate the amount of proteins excreted in a day. The American College of Rheumatology requires the presence of 0.5 gm of protein in the urine over a 24 hour period to meet the criteria for diagnosing what is called *proteinuria*. Patients with cellular casts may also have other types of casts, including the following:

- Red blood cells casts
- Hemoglobin casts

- Mixed-elements casts
- Tubular casts
- Granular casts.

If kidney involvement is diagnosed, a kidney biopsy is recommended to determine the extent of the disease or damage to the kidneys. The degree of damage determines which of the six types (classifications) of kidney disease the patient has and which type of treatment will follow.

To understand the classification, it is important to know how the kidneys work. The kidneys are reddish brown, bean-shaped organs that lie on either side of the spinal column in the back of the abdomen. The filtering devices of the blood, the kidneys remove waste products from the body by excreting them in urine. The kidneys also control the amount of red blood cell formation by secreting a hormone called *erythropoietin* and an enzyme called *renin* to help regulate blood pressure. Essentially, the kidneys help balance the concentration and volume of body fluids.

The kidneys receive oxygenated blood through the renal arteries, as shown in Figure 3a. Once they enter the kidneys, the arteries divide into branches in the different sections of each kidney (like a trunk develops into a tree by producing multiple branches of different sizes.) One of these branches leads to the formation of *nephrons*, the functional sections of the kidney. The renal vein transports blood, with wastes, out of the kidneys, and the rest of the wastes are excreted from body through the urine, which passes through the *ureters* to the bladder and then to the urethra (see Figure 3a).

The kidneys contain around one million nephrons, each of which consists of a renal *corpuscle* and a renal *tubule*. The renal corpuscle is a collection or cluster of blood capillaries (the smallest blood vessels in the body) called the *glomerulus* (a group of small blood vessels in the kidney responsible for filtering waste from the blood), which is covered by a capsule. As seen in Figure 3a, the renal tubule looks like a net and has a knot, which is the glomerulus. The renal tubule is responsible for water balance, electrolyte regulation, and the discharge of waste out of the kidneys and the body. Other structures of the kidney are also involved in the normal functioning and fluid balance of the body.

Let's look at the six classifications for kidney disease in lupus that may interrupt the normal function or structure of the kidneys. The classifications are based on criteria used by the World Health Organization (WHO).

Figure 3a. Anatomy of the Kidneys

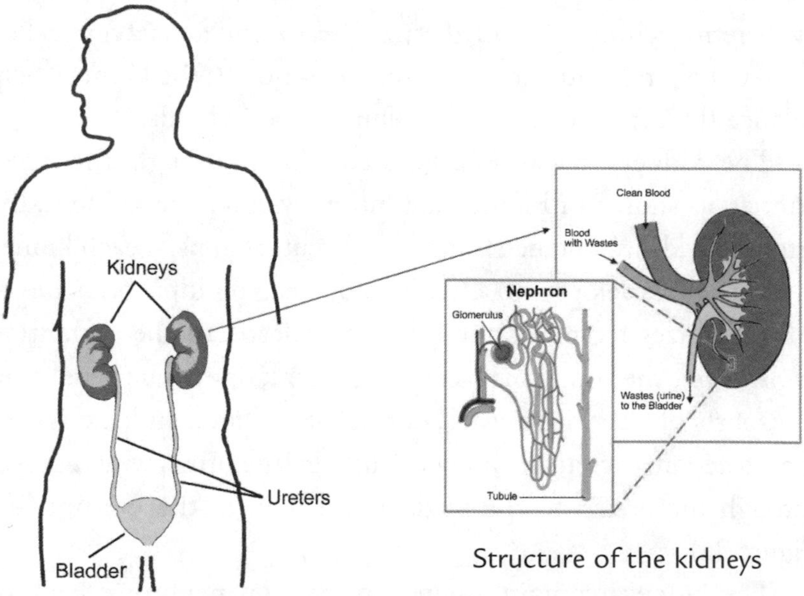

Location of the kidneys in the body. Note that they have a shape of a bean.

Structure of the kidneys

Figure 3b. Normal Glomerular Capillary

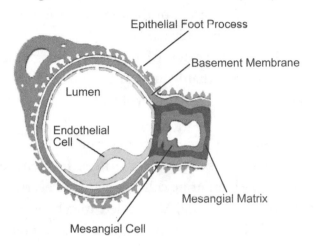

- *Class I:* The patient may have excessive amounts of protein in the urine (*proteinuria*) but not display any abnormal changes of the kidney.
- *Class II:* There is minimal change or damage to the kidneys in a part of the glomerulus called the *mesangial* area. This damage results in an increased number of mesangial cells (Figure 3b).
- *Class III:* This is known as *focal proliferative lupus nephritis*. It may indicate more damage in the mesangial area and progressive damage to other areas of the kidneys. Further damage may include *necrosis* or death of cells in some areas, and infiltration of *leukocytes* (white blood cells) in some sections of the glomerulus. It is called focal because not all the glomerulus is affected and the damage exists only in small areas.
- *Class IV:* In this stage, the changes involve more than 50 percent of the glomerular surface and cause extensive damage to the kidney.

- *Class V:* The changes involve the membrane covering the glomerulus. The surface of the capillary walls—that are otherwise smooth—thicken.
- *Class VI:* There are extensive changes of the glomerulus known as *sclerosis* (hardening) of the glomeruli. The damage at this stage is irreversible.

Kidney disease in lupus patients can be monitored with routine laboratory tests. Some of the most frequent tests are a urine sample, a 24-hour urine collection at least every six months (in patients with proteinuria), a complete metabolic panel (which evaluates blood chemistry, enzymes, and kidney function), and immunologic tests.

Urinalysis can indicate the presence and severity of kidney disease. For example, proteinuria, detected in repeated samples of urine, can be an early indicator of kidney disease. The presence of red blood cells (RBCs), white blood cells (WBCs), and cellular casts in the urine are other indicators of kidney disease. A 24-hour urine sample is often ordered to measure how quickly *creatinine* (a chemical waste by-product of muscle metabolism) is removed from the body when kidney disease is suspected. This test measures the glomerular filtration rate (GFR), which is a measurement of the efficiency of the kidneys in filtering blood to excrete metabolic waste.

The kidneys may be damaged by another complication of lupus, called *lupus nephritis*. In this condition, the kidneys do not excrete creatinine efficiently. This inability results in abnormal kidney function and can further damage the kidneys. The doctor may order a kidney biopsy at this point to determine the degree of damage to the kidney. In addition, patients with kidney disease are given specific immunologic tests such as an anti-double-stranded DNA (anti-ds DNA) test (explained later in this chapter), a *complement* test (C3, C4, CH50), and the ENA panel (which includes the anti-P and anti-nRNP) to test the strength of the immune system.

Complements are proteins in the blood that combine with antibodies to destroy foreign cells, or antigens. Complement proteins also cause blood vessels to become dilated and "leaky" causing redness and swelling during an inflammatory response. There are twelve complement components in the blood, each identified by numbers. Each complement has sub-components that are further identified by letters of the alphabet. In lupus, there is a deficiency of some of the complements giving rise to a condition called *hypocomplementemia*. The most frequently absent (usually due to genetic causes) complements are: C1 (C1q, C1s, and C1r), C2, C3, and C4. Complements C3 and C4 are usually decreased in patients with active kidney disease. Individuals with a complete deficiency of complement component C1q have over a 90 percent probability of developing lupus. Complement C2, at a frequency of about one in ten thousand persons, is the most common of the lupus-associated deficiencies and approximately 75 percent of patients with C4 deficiency develop lupus. Complements C4 and CH50 (or total hemolytic complement) can be decreased prior to a lupus flare-up. A CH50 blood test is used to measure deficiencies of the complement system and is routinely administered to lupus patients as a means of evaluating complement levels.

Treatment for kidney disease may include immunosuppressive therapies such as corticosteroids, chemotherapy, and dialysis in the later stages of kidney disease. The specific treatment will vary from patient to patient (see Chapter 6). Today, most patients with kidney disease respond well to therapy, thus preventing complete kidney failure. Ongoing research and clinical trials seek to discover new therapies that have fewer side effects and are more effective in shorter periods of time.

SEROSITIS

Serositis is the general term used to describe an inflammation of the lining of the heart or lungs. When it involves the heart lining it is called *pericarditis*, and in the lungs it is called *pleurisy*. Pleurisy is common in lupus patients. The pleura or *serous* coat is a shiny, thin, transparent membrane that covers each lung. The pleural membranes prevent the lungs from making direct contact with the chest wall and the diaphragm. The inner or *visceral* layer of the pleura is attached to the lungs, and the outer or parietal layer is attached to the chest wall. Both layers are covered with mesothelial cells, which secrete a small amount of fluid that provides lubrication between the chest wall and the lungs. The layers are held in place by a film of pleural fluid, similar to two glass microscope slides that are wetted and then stuck together. The pleural membranes prevent the lungs from making direct contact with the chest wall and diaphragm. Cells in the pleural space are primarily *mesothelial* cells that line the surfaces of the pleural membranes and some white blood cells. The pleural membranes are semipermeable, that is, they allow fluid to pass through them. A small amount of fluid continuously seeps out of the blood vessels through the parietal pleura. The visceral pleura absorb fluid, which then drains into the lymphatic system (that collects and filters all the body's waste) and then returns to the blood.

Protein in the circulation and balanced pressures keep excessive amounts of fluid from seeping out of the blood vessels into the pleural space. Under normal conditions, pleural fluid is formed in small amounts to lubricate the surfaces of the pleura.

Pleurisy can result in an abnormal amount of pleural fluid collecting in the lungs. This condition is called *pleural effusion*. Under pathological or disease conditions, two types of effusions can develop: *transudative* and *exudative* pleural effusions.

Transudative pleural effusions are usually caused by a problem in the normal pressure in the lung. Congestive heart failure is the most common cause of transudative effusion. Exudative effusions form as a result of inflammation (irritation and swelling) of the pleura and is often caused by lung disease. Some of the diseases that can cause exudative pleural effusions are collagen-vascular diseases (such as lupus), cancer, pneumonia, tuberculosis and other lung infections, drug reactions, asbestosis, and sarcoidosis (an inflammatory disease). Exudative pleural effusion can also cause chest pains and inflammation of the lungs.

During a physical examination, your physician will listen to the sound of your breathing with a stethoscope and may tap on your chest to listen for dullness, which could be produced by fluid retention in the chest. A diagnosis is confirmed by noting changes in the chest X-ray. The type of effusion can be diagnosed by taking a sample of the fluid by a procedure called *thoracentesis*. In this procedure, fluid is removed via a needle inserted between the ribs into the chest cavity, while the patient is under a local anesthetic.

Pericarditis is the most common sign of heart involvement in lupus. It can occur at any time during the course of the disease, but sometimes it may be the first identifiable symptom. Patients experience pain in the anterior or back of the chest, and the neck, back, or arms. The pain worsens when lying down and generally improves when the patient sits up. There may be shortness of breath, rapid heartbeat, swelling of the legs, fever, and an abnormal heart sound called a "friction rub." Pleurisy with or without pleural effusion may also be present with pericarditis. The pericarditis episodes can be isolated or can repeat throughout the course of the disease. It is diagnosed through the patient's history, a physical exam, a chest X-ray, and by noting changes in the heartbeat as measured by an electrocardiogram (EKG). An echocardiogram (a sonogram of the heart) demonstrates the heart's blood flow and helps the doctor evaluate heart function to determine if fluid has collected in the sac of the heart.

Treatment may vary depending on the patient's specific symptoms. In mild cases, nonsteroidal anti-inflammatory drugs can be given to alleviate pain. In other cases, corticosteroids can be given. Usually, chest X-rays are repeated to evaluate how well the heart and lungs are responding to treatment. (Further details of disease treatment follow in Chapter 6.)

NEUROLOGIC CONDITIONS

Lupus may also affect the brain and nervous system. Neurologic conditions (conditions that involve the brain and nerves) are present when a patient experiences seizures (convulsions) or psychosis unrelated to any other disease, medication, or drugs. Up to 60 percent of adults, and 40 percent of children with lupus may display symptoms of *neuropsychiatric* lupus.

Seizures occur in up to 20 percent of lupus patients. They may occur simultaneously with the diagnosis or during a flare-up of the disease. Several types of seizure patterns can occur, but the *grand mal* or *tonic-clonic* seizures during which the patient loses consciousness are the most common. In rare instances, some lupus patients may have repeated, multiple seizures within in a short period of time. These types of seizures are called *status epilepticus seizures.*

Psychotic complications develop more frequently in adults than in children. A psychotic patient may display psychoses in different ways. The patient can be calm or agitated, passive or aggressively violent, or withdrawn. Some patients feel as though they are removed from their own body, and some may even be homicidal or suicidal.

Patients may also display the following neurologic conditions:

- *Hallucination:* The hallucinating patient has a flawed perception of objective reality. The patient may think he or she is seeing, hearing, touching, tasting, or smelling something not really there.
- *Illusional thinking:* In illusional thinking, the patient misinterprets information about a real object and combines it with a mental image to create a false perception of the object or the situation.
- *Delusional thinking:* The patient suffering from delusional thinking has an irrational or false belief that cannot be altered by a rational argument.

If the patient appears depressed and *grandiose*, that is, he or she has an exaggerated opinion of himself or herself that has no realistic basis, he or she may be given the diagnosis of *psychotic depression*, or *mania* with psychotic symptoms. This type of psychosis is called a *functional* disorder, because the patient complains of symptoms for which no physical cause can be found. By contrast, if the patient displays panic and anxiety, along with psychotic disorientation, an *organic* or physical disorder may be the cause. In cases where there might be damage or changes in an internal organ of the body, further evaluation is often needed to diagnose the underlying cause of the psychotic behavior.

Some patients can display symptoms of *delirium*, an acute disorder of mental processes caused by brain disease. Delirium can take the form of illusions, disorientation, hallucinations, or increased excitement. Lupus can cause delirium if the brain is affected as can infections or other degenerative conditions. In the early stages, delirium can present as disorientation, agitation, increased excitement, and sleep disturbances. Patients can develop or display a sudden change of mental disturbance within a day, which is often characteristic for the diagnosis.

Treatment for lupus-related seizures can include anticonvulsant drugs or immunosuppressive therapy, depending on the symptoms of the patient. The treatment for psychotic disorders will depend on the type of disorder and symptoms present at the time of diagnosis. In cases where neuropsychiatric lupus is suspected, it is extremely important that the correct diagnosis be made in order to exclude any other potential causes of neuropsychiatric disease such as infections, medications, metabolic or other medical disorders, or psychiatric conditions.

HEMATOLOGIC DISORDERS

Hematologic or blood disorder is present when the blood cells and the coagulation (clotting) pathways are affected. The patient's white blood cells and platelets (cells that prevent bleeding) may be decreased, or the patient may display *hemolytic anemia*, a condition in which red blood cells are destroyed faster than they can be replaced. These abnormal conditions are detected by blood tests.

White blood cells protect us against infection. There are many different types of white blood cells. A reduction in the number of white blood cells can be the result of disease, complications, or adverse reaction to medication. For these reasons, frequent blood tests are a routine part of the follow-up of a lupus patient. The test is commonly known as a CBC (cell blood count) test.

Low white blood cell counts usually occur in up to 90 percent of patients with active or severe disease. When the white blood cell count is low, patients are more likely to develop infections. There are two types of white blood cell count conditions that are of particular importance to the lupus patient: *lymphopenia* and *leukopenia.*

Lymphopenia is the condition in which there is an abnormally low number of lymphocytes (a white blood cell involved in the immune system) in the blood. It occurs frequently independently of *leukopenia* (described below), but the two conditions may occur together in lupus patients.

Leukopenia, a decrease in the number of circulating white blood cells, occurs in up to 50 percent of lupus patients at some time during the course of the disease and is generally mild. Lupus patients of sub-Saharan African heritage may naturally have a low level of leukocytes (cells that help the body to fight infections and other disease) due to their genetic heritage. Both lymphopenia and leucopenia can be caused by the chemotherapy drugs used in lupus therapy, and activation of the disease itself, but both conditions respond to treatment with immunosuppressive therapy such as corticosteroids.

Thrombocytopenia is a decrease in the number of platelets in the blood. It can result in small red dots in the skin (*petechiae*) and excessive bruising and bleeding. In lupus, serious organ involvement is associated with thrombocytopenia. This includes neuropsychiatric manifestations, hemolytic anemia, *antiphospholipid syndrome*, an immune system disorder characterized by excessive clotting of the blood, and kidney disease. Most patients with mild to moderate cases of thrombocytopenia do not need any specific therapy. Those patients that require therapy usually respond to an immunosuppressive course of treatment. In extreme cases of bleeding with incomplete response to therapy, removal of the spleen may be indicated.

Hemolytic anemia is caused by a decrease in the red blood cells caused by early (premature) destruction of red blood cells by the body's own antibodies. This is frequently referred to as *hemolysis*. Ordinarily, red blood cells have a life span of approximately 90–120 days, at which time the old cells are destroyed and replaced by the body's natural processes. In patients with hemolytic anemia, the cells are broken down at a faster rate than the bone marrow can produce new cells. It occurs in at least 10–15 percent of lupus patients, though it is more common in women and may affect any age group. In up to 6 percent of the time, hemolytic anemia can be the initial manifestation of lupus. The condition usually starts suddenly, with typical symptoms of anemia such as fatigue and paleness of the skin.

Treatment should be initiated immediately after diagnosis. Immunosuppressive therapy will vary depending on the different complications present in each case. It is important that patients with low platelets or bleeding problems notify their doctors if they are taking aspirin or nonsteroidal anti-inflammatory drugs because these medications can worsen the condition.

IMMUNOLOGIC DISORDERS

Immunologic disorders—disorders of the immune system—are diagnosed through blood tests for abnormal antibodies. Normally, the immune system makes proteins called antibodies to protect the body against foreign invaders such as viruses, bacteria, and other harmful agents. These invaders are called *antigens*. The body responds to antigens by making antibodies to attack them.

In lupus, the immune system loses its ability to differentiate between antigens and its own cells, resulting in a production of antibodies known as *autoantibodies*. Some of the immunologic abnormalities in lupus are the presence of anti-double-stranded DNA, anti-Smith (anti-Sm) antibody, *anticardiolipin* (a condition characterized by clots in the arteries and the veins) antibodies, a false-positive syphilis test, and complement deficiency. These autoantibodies can set disease processes in motion that can cause inflammation, pain, and injury to the body's tissues.

Anti-double-stranded DNA is present in 60–80 percent of adult lupus patients, in almost all children with active lupus, and its presence is associated with kidney disease. Higher concentrations or *titers* of anti-double-stranded DNA are seen with lupus flare-ups, and decreased concentrations usually result with adequate treatment. Anti-double-stranded DNA antibodies are found almost exclusively in lupus patients, but a small number of patients with other diseases show lower titers as well.

Anti-Smith antibody is another type of protein found primarily in lupus patients but is only present in 30 percent of the cases. Anti-Smith can occur together with another antibody called anti-U1 RNP and relates to disease of the central nervous system. Anti-Smith antibodies are more frequently present in African-American patients than in white lupus patients.

Complements, as discussed earlier in the chapter, are a group of proteins that help protect the body from invading organisms. The complement system is composed of proteins that activate the immune complex system. Any alteration in any of the complements leads to abnormalities in the functioning of the immune system. Hence, examination of total serum complement is one of the laboratory tests given to a patient with active lupus. Measurement of CH50 (total hemolytic complement) is frequently tested in lupus patients to evaluate the integrity and to identify any deficiencies of the entire complement system. Genetic deficiencies of complements C1q, C2, and C4 are rare but are commonly associated with lupus. Complements C3 and C4 are commonly measured in lupus patients and are associated with kidney involvement. When the disease is active, the complement levels decrease. Normal levels are obtained after treatment of lupus flare-ups.

Antiphospholipid antibodies are present in up to 40 percent of lupus patients. Antiphospholipid antibody syndrome is a disorder of the immune system characterized by excessive clotting of blood, complications of pregnancy including miscarriages, unexplained fetal death, premature birth, *hemolytic anemia* in which blood cells are destroyed faster than they can be replaced, and reduced blood platelet counts (*thrombocytopenia*). Antiphospholipid antibody syndrome occurs in up to 15 percent of lupus patients.

The *antinuclear antibody test*, or ANA test, is frequently positive in lupus patients. In fact, a positive antinuclear antibody test, unrelated to any other disease or medication, occurs in approximately 95 percent of lupus patients. However, a positive antinuclear antibody test is not specific for lupus because a positive reaction can occur in people without lupus who may or may not have any other type of disease. Spouses and family members of lupus patients can have a positive antinuclear antibody test without having lupus. There are four patterns of ANA antibodies—*speckled, homogeneous, nucleolar*, and *cytoplasmic*.

In otherwise healthy patients, a weak positive antinuclear antibody test does not meet the criteria for lupus; further testing is not necessary and is not generally seen as a cause for concern. However, if there is a positive antinuclear antibody titer with some symptoms or other laboratory tests suggest lupus, periodic retesting and follow-up exams are advisable as some of these patients may develop lupus over time. Patients with a negative antinuclear antibody test will have other antibodies in their blood in addition to other criteria to aid the doctor in making the diagnosis of lupus.

CHAPTER FOUR

>~

OTHER PRESENTATIONS

CAROLYN'S STORY

For me, living with lupus has not been as bad as it has for others. I was diagnosed in 1980 at the age of thirty-four after a very high fever and what I thought was the flu. Until 1985, when I had my only child, I was not on medication, nor did I have any symptoms. But in my sixth month of pregnancy, I developed a condition called "placentia previa" which made me hemorrhage. I was told that I would have to spend the remainder of the pregnancy in the hospital; I was forbidden to get out of bed. I was not allowed to sit up except to eat, and even then I had to be at a forty-five degree angle. I was very uncomfortable because it was July and one of the hottest summers on record. My night sweats were so bad the nurses called me their thermostat! When I went into the hospital I weighed 116 pounds and the day before I delivered I had lost two more pounds. I was getting 3,000 calories a day and still could not gain weight. In my seventh month, my daughter was born prematurely. Thank the Lord, *she was breathing on her own without any problems. I found that the prednisone the doctor prescribed worked well for me. For two years I had no symptoms and was fine until my daughter developed asthma and was in and out of the hospital with pneumonia. I was working a very demanding work schedule at an accounting firm and, as a result of all this stress, my lupus flared. I developed a severe rash from my face and arms down to my abdomen. Finally, because I was so tired all the time and felt like I was going to have a nervous breakdown, I quit the job I'd had for eight years to stay home with my daughter.*

A month after my stressful schedule ended, the rash went away and I was once again symptom-free. I have been on prednisone ever since and only occasionally experience joint pain—which is usually caused by not taking my medicine.

➶

Along with the symptoms discussed in previous chapters, a patient with lupus may experience a number of others. Symptoms such as fatigue; fever; weight loss; hair loss; enlarged lymph nodes; general weakness; Raynaud's phenomenon, a condition that affects blood vessels in the hands and feet; and other skin rashes may occur before the diagnosis of lupus is made. Because these symptoms are so common in other conditions, including infections, it is extremely important for your physician to perform a complete evaluation to rule out other disease. Your physician may perform several radiological and laboratory tests to confirm your diagnosis.

Fatigue is usually one of the first and most common symptoms in patients with active lupus or an impending flare-up. It is also present as a result of other conditions, such as depression, infections, or sleep disturbances. Fatigue can be one of the most common, debilitating symptoms in lupus and may cause disruption in the patient's lifestyle. Patients usually describe the fatigue as "flu-like" because of limited energy and little desire to perform their usual daily activities. The fatigue caused by lupus usually responds to corticosteroid therapy. (Detailed therapy information follows in Chapter 6.)

Fever in lupus patients may be one of the first symptoms of a flare-up. Fever is present in up to 70–100 percent of lupus patients, especially in children. Fevers can be as high as 102°F and last for a few days at a time. Some patients may even spike a fever higher than 102°F. Fever is said to be secondary to lupus when other causes, such as infections, are ruled out. The fevers occur at any time of the day or night, as opposed to following any specific pattern as seen in other diseases. The fever in lupus patients usually responds well to corticosteroid therapy.

Weight loss in lupus patients is usually caused by loss of appetite (anorexia) which happens up to 71 percent of the time in adults and 35 percent in children. Patients may feel so weak that they have no energy to even get up in the mornings, eat, and perform their daily activities. Patients may lose 10 percent of their total body weight; children with lupus may lose even more. Weight loss is usually resolved with disease treatment, namely corticosteroids, which helps increase the appetite. Patients who continue to lose weight even after the disease has been treated need further evaluation for poor intake, disorders of the metabolic system, or malignancies (rarely seen in lupus).

Hair loss (alopecia) can occur in children and adults before the diagnosis of lupus and during a flare-up. Patients may notice an increased loss of hair while brushing or on the pillow after a night's sleep. In general, there is thinning or patchy hair loss and the texture of the hair may be altered, but total hair loss does not occur. The hair above the forehead becomes brittle and can break off easily, leaving short hairs at the hairline. In some patients hair loss may be caused by medications, such as the chemotherapy drugs that are sometimes prescribed to treat lupus.

Enlarged lymph nodes (lymphadenopathy) frequently appear at some time during the course of the disease in children, usually in the neck area or in the underarm area. In some cases the lymph nodes can be extremely enlarged and may be confused with a malignancy. Yet malignancies are very rare in children with lupus. On occasion, enlarged lymph nodes may be accompanied by a mild enlargement of the spleen (splenomegaly). Enlarged lymph nodes usually resolve or go away over time, but flare-ups with active disease may occur.

Muscle weakness (myositis) and muscle pain (myalgia) are other common manifestations in lupus patients but are especially common in children. Found in 50 percent of the cases, this inflammation, caused by muscle enzymes, can be measured by a blood test. Some 3–5 percent of these patients will have an increase in muscle enzymes such as *creatine phosphokinase* (CPK), an enzyme found predominantly in the heart, brain, and skeletal muscle. Muscle involvement is usually short term and responds to the therapy given in active disease.

Myasthenia gravis, an autoimmune neuromuscular disease characterized by varying degrees of weakness of the skeletal (voluntary) muscles of the body, is rare but can occur in a small number of lupus patients. In myasthenia gravis, antibodies block, alter, or destroy the receptors for *acetylcholine* (an important neurotransmitter) and prevent the muscle from contracting. Acetylcholine is a substance found in nerve fibers that transmits impulses throughout the body. Patients with myasthenia gravis have specific muscle weakness but not generalized fatigue.

Problems with eye movement such as *ptosis* (drooping of the eyelid) or *diplopia* (double vision) are the initial symptoms of myasthenia gravis in two-thirds of patients; almost all develop both symptoms within two years. Weakness in the muscles in the back of the throat causes difficulty chewing, swallowing, or talking and is the initial symptom in one-sixth of patients. Limb weakness is seen in only 10 percent. Initial weakness is rarely limited to single muscle groups such as the neck or fingers or hips. The severity of weakness fluctuates during the day, usually being least severe in the morning and worsening as the day progresses, especially after prolonged use of the affected muscles.

The course of *myasthenia gravis* varies but is usually progressive, that is, it tends to get worse over time. In 10 percent of cases, however, the weakness is restricted to the muscles of the eye. The other 90 percent experience progressive weakness during the first two years, which may involve the oropharyngeal (mouth and throat) and limb muscles. Maximum weakness occurs during the first year in two-thirds of patients. In one study, one-third improved spontaneously, one-third became worse, and one-third died of the disease. Spontaneous improvement frequently occurs early in the course of the disease. Symptoms may fluctuate over a relatively short period of time and then become progressively more severe for several years (active stage). The active stage is usually followed by an inactive state during which fluctuations in strength still occur but are attributable to fatigue, intermittent illness, or other factors. After several years, the weakness often levels off and the most severely involved muscles become *atrophic* (burnt-out).

Factors that worsen myasthenia gravis symptoms are stress, systemic illness (especially viral respiratory infections), hypothyroidism or hyperthyroidism (problems associated with the thyroid gland), pregnancy, the menstrual cycle, drugs affecting neuromuscular transmission (muscle movement), and increases in body temperature. Treatment goals must be individualized according to the severity of disease and the patient's age, sex, and degree of functional impairment. A patient's response to any form of treatment will depend completely on the severity of the symptoms and disease activity.

Raynaud's phenomenon can be present in patients with lupus and is usually triggered by cold or emotional stress. Raynaud's phenomenon is frequently seen in children and adults and it is more common in women than in men. Raynaud's can be present prior to the diagnosis of lupus, but there are many causes for this disorder so a diagnosis of Raynaud's syndrome by itself does not mean that a patient will develop lupus. In other words, many patients with only Raynaud's phenomenon may never develop lupus. These patients are said to have *idiopathic* Raynaud's phenomenon.

The diagnosis of Raynaud's phenomenon is made by physical examination and by the patient's history. Patients may notice a change of color of the tips of the fingers and/or toes to white, blue, or red. This transformation corresponds to closing of the blood vessels and *cyanosis* (lack of oxygen), which causes bluish discoloration of the skin and mucous membranes.

Vasospasm (a sudden closure of the blood vessels limiting blood flow to an area) may lead to numbness or tingling of the fingers or toes. The skin in the affected area may eventually become stiff with *sclerodactyly*, a localized thickening of the skin and tightness of the fingers and toes, or *atrophy* (wasting) of the soft tissue of the hands and feet. As a result, ulcers may form in the affected area of the fingers or toes and become progressively worse, leading to gangrene and *necrosis* (death of the tissue). This phenomenon occurs in a small number of patients and can also involve the nose, ears, and lips. For this reason, it is very important for patients with Raynaud's phenomenon to protect their hands and feet from the cold by warming the area gently with their own body heat or warm water and wearing warmer clothing.

Other preventive treatments for Raynaud's disease include behavioral changes, such as smoking cessation (nicotine affects skin temperature and constricts blood vessels), reducing stress, and exercising. Medications used for Raynaud's disease include calcium channel blockers, alpha blockers, and nitroglycerin.

Other types of *skin rash* can be present in lupus patients. One of these is *livedo reticularis*, which has the appearance of a purplish lace-like pattern on the arms or legs. This type of rash is also seen in patients with *antiphospholipid antibody syndrome* (see Chapter 3). Patients can also have *lupus panniculitis* (also known as *lupus profundus*), which is the result of an inflammatory process in the fat under the skin or in the tissues of the deep skin layer. This inflammation leads to firm, deep *nodules* (small masses) or patches of skin that are different in appearance and feel from the rest of the surrounding area.

Other skin manifestations that may be present in lupus include *urticaria* (itch), *bullous* (blistering), and *angioedema* (swelling in small areas under the skin). Remember that these symptoms can be present in diseases other than lupus, and not all of these symptoms are exhibited in every lupus patient.

CHAPTER FIVE

)❧

COMPLICATIONS

L UPUS PATIENTS CAN develop several complications during
the course of their disease. Some of these complications
can be life threatening and require early and aggressive
treatment. As mentioned before, every patient will have unique
and unpredictable symptoms. We cannot know in advance which
person will respond to a specific therapy or which complications
will develop. Each patient must be treated on an individual basis.

THE SKIN

Lupus, as we have seen, can affect any organ in the body, resulting
in a variety of complications. Discoid lupus, which affects only
the skin, can convert into systemic lupus in 5–10 percent of cases.
Lupus nephritis, an inflammation of the kidney, is usually the first
sign that the patient has developed the systemic type of lupus.
Once this occurs, the change is irreversible and other organ
involvement and treatments will follow the same course as for
those patients who had an initial diagnosis of systemic lupus.

Another skin complication is *skin vasculitis*, an inflammation of the small blood vessels in the skin. Occurring in up to 70 percent of lupus patients, skin vasculitis can affect patients of all ages and gender. Skin vasculitis can start as an itchy rash, *petechiae* (small purple or pinkish dots), skin ulcers, or painful *nodules* (hard masses) and can lead to a condition called *leukocytoclastic vasculitis*. This diagnosis is made by skin biopsy through a procedure called a *punch biopsy*. An itchy rash is often the initial skin manifestation of lupus in some patients. The rash usually responds to the same corticosteroid therapy used to treat active disease. As suspected in other lupus-related inflammation of the lower extremities, the production of antiphospholipid antibodies (see Chapter 3: Hematologic Disorders) may be the reason for skin ulcers.

Telangiectasias are dilated superficial blood vessels and is another common type of skin vasculitis in lupus. It involves a prolonged dilatation or inflammation of a group of capillaries in the skin, causing elevated, dark red blotches. They are usually small and located close to the nail fold in old lupus skin lesions, or less frequently, on the fingers, palms, or face. In addition, some patients may have dilatation of the nail fold capillaries. These lesions are also seen in other autoimmune diseases, so their presence alone does not determine a lupus diagnosis.

Other less frequently reported skin conditions seen in lupus patients are:

- *Erythema multiforme* (EM), which are eruptions of small, flat, red *macules* or spots that sometimes have blistered areas in the center.
- *Papules*, small, solid and usually cone-shaped elevations of the skin that often occur in clusters.

- *Cutaneous mucinosis*, a build-up of abnormal amounts of *mucin*, a thick, clear, sticky fluid under the skin.
- Pigmentation changes, *anetoderma* (skin damage resulting in wrinkles), *cutis laxa* (loss of elasticity of the skin), *lichen planus* (flat-topped reddish-purplish bumps that often have an angular shape), and *acanthosis nigricans* (velvety, light-brown to black, pigmentation usually on the neck, under the arms, or in the groin).

EYES

The eyes can be affected by lupus in a variety of ways. Think of the eye as a hollow, fluid-filled ball made up of three layers, where the tough outer layer is the *sclera*, the middle layer is the *uvea*, and the innermost layer is the retina. Patients may develop inflammation of the front or back area of the eye (see Figure 4). Some lupus patients may develop *uveitis*, an inflammation of any of the structures in the middle portion of the eye.

Another complication is *retinal vasculitis*, an inflammation of the vessels that supply blood to the retina. Ten percent of patients

Figure 4. The Anatomy of the Eye

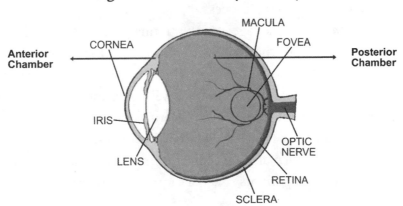

will develop *episcleritis*, an inflammation of the *sclera*, or *optic neuritis*, an inflammation of the optic nerve.

The patient with episcleritis may not know it immediately because he or she may not experience any symptoms or pain. There is usually redness in one or both eyes however. There may also be a translucent white nodule within the inflamed area (*nodular episcleritis*). Most cases of episcleritis will go away on their own, though patients experiencing discomfort may benefit from topical anti-inflammatory agents and lubricants. A 1 percent solution of *prednisolone* acetate or *fluorometholone acetate*, applied three to four times during the day, will generally speed healing and decrease tenderness. The patient may use cold compresses and lubricating eye drops if discomfort persists. In more severe cases, as in nodular episcleritis, oral nonsteroidal anti-inflammatory drugs may be required to reduce the inflammation.

Optic neuritis, an inflammation of the optic nerve, may cause sudden, partial loss of vision in the affected eye. The patient may also experience loss of vision in one eye, loss of color vision, or pain upon eye movement, or the pupil of the affected eye may not constrict or narrow normally in bright light, leading to a condition known as *photophobia*. Though normal vision returns within two to three weeks without treatment, corticosteroids can be used to accelerate the process.

Retinopathy, or damage to the retina, is present in lupus patients 7 percent of the time, with deposits in the liquid part of the eye called "cotton-wool" spots that may be accompanied by hemorrhage (bleeding), *papilledema* (swelling of the optic disc), or *occlusion* (blockage) of the optic vein. Retinal damage can also occur as a complication of the anti-malarial therapy used frequently in treatment. The anti-malarial medication most commonly used in treating lupus patients is Plaquenil® (generic name, hydroxychloroquine). This drug is a relatively mild treatment and is intended for long-term control of disease. Retinal damage caused by the use of anti-malarial therapy is dose related, and most cases of eye disease occur in patients receiving more than 400 mg of Plaquenil®, or more than 250 mg of Aralen® (chloroquine phosphate), another anti-malarial drug, daily. Retinal damage caused by the use of Plaquenil® is sometimes reversible if it is treated early. However, damage caused by Aralen® is irreversible.

Lupus complications in the eye are rare, but patients need to have an initial examination performed by an ophthalmologist before starting therapy and follow-up exams every six months thereafter. On many occasions, the ophthalmologist can detect minor changes in the retinal pigment that indicate early damage due to the use of anti-malarial drugs. In addition to tests of visual acuity and eye pressure, regular eye checkups may be needed to test color vision and the visual field to check if the patient has developed "blind spots."

Some lupus patients may develop a condition known as *xerostomia*, which can be a symptom of another disease, *Sjögren's syndrome*, which also affects some lupus patients. These patients experience dryness and the sensation of sand in the eye, redness of the *conjunctiva* (the thin, transparent tissue that covers the outer surface of the eye), and sensitivity to light. This condition can be diagnosed by a test called the Schirmer's test, which uses a specialized filter paper to measure the amount of tears produced by the eye. A positive test is obtained when there is a decrease in the amount of tears produced. Another test that can be done uses specially formulated dyes that can help to detect scarring and dry areas of the eye.

Patients with xerostomia may also have inflammation of the glands that produce saliva, resulting in a decreased production of saliva, which then produces swelling of the *parotid* gland (a gland situated near the ear). Such swelling may be painful and can result in difficulty in chewing and swallowing, abnormalities of taste, severe dental cavities, and strong breath smell (halitosis). The diagnosis can be confirmed by detecting abnormal changes of the gland or a biopsy of a small portion of the salivary gland from the lower lip.

Sjögren's syndrome, a condition that affects some lupus patients, is an autoimmune disease in which the patient's white blood cells attack the glands that produce moisture throughout the body. Patients diagnosed with Sjögren's syndrome may experience dryness in the nose, throat, and vagina. Patients with Sjögren's syndrome usually have a positive blood test for the presence of the anti-Ro (anti-SSA) and anti-La (anti-SSB) antibodies. Anti-Ro antibodies can be correlated with ANA-negative lupus, Sjögren's syndrome, and antiphospholipid antibodies. Anti-La occurs in patients with, as well as some lupus patients without, Sjogren's syndrome.

Dryness of the eyes can also occur as a side effect of several medications that mimic the drying effect of Sjögren's syndrome. Such medications include certain sleep disturbance and anxiety disorder medicines, painkillers, antidepressants, antihistamines, and muscle relaxants. Patients with lupus and other autoimmune diseases frequently use these medications; therefore dryness of the eyes does not always confirm a diagnosis of Sjögren's syndrome.

CARDIOVASCULAR SYSTEM

Lungs

Patients with pleurisy may have a condition known as *pleural effusion*, which is a build-up of fluid in the lung cavity. Pleural effusion causes pain and difficulty with deep breathing. The patient with a pleural effusion will take shallow, superficial breaths upon minor exertion. Pleural effusion occurs when the inflammatory process disrupts the normal functioning of the lung. The patient may experience a sensation of not getting enough air. This can result in chest tightness, pressure, or chest discomfort.

In normal breathing, we inhale air through the nose or mouth; the air then travels down the trachea to the bronchus, where it first enters the lung (see Figure 5). The air goes through the bronchi, into the even smaller bronchioles, and last into the alveoli. Our lungs bring fresh oxygen into our bodies and remove carbon dioxide and other gaseous waste products. As we breathe air in, we use the muscles of our rib cage and especially the diaphragm to pull air into our lungs. As we inhale, the diaphragm contracts or tightens and flattens, allowing air to be sucked into

Figure 5. The Respiratory System

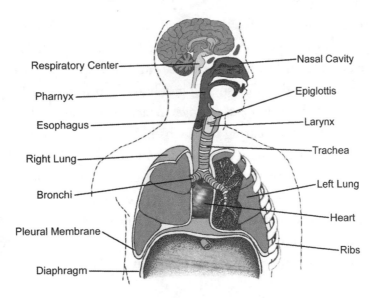

the lungs. The diaphragm and the rib cage muscles relax, and air is removed from the body; the muscles do no work when we breathe out.

When we inhale through the nose or the mouth, the mucous membranes warm and moisten the air and trap particles of foreign matter. The air containing the oxygen our bodies need passes through the throat into the trachea or windpipe. The trachea divides into the left and right bronchi. Like a tree branch, each bronchus divides again and again, becoming narrower and narrower. The smallest airways end in the *alveoli*, which are small, thin air sacs arranged in clusters like bunches of balloons or bunches of grapes on stems. When we breathe in by enlarging the chest cage, the "balloons" expand as air rushes in to fill the vacuum. When we breathe out, the "balloons" relax and air moves out of the lungs. Tiny blood vessels surround each of the 300 million alveoli in the lungs. Oxygen moves across the walls of the air sacs, where it is picked up by the blood and carried to the rest of the body. Carbon dioxide passes into the air sacs from the blood and is breathed out.

Healthy lungs have effective ways to keep clean. Mucus in the airways traps dirt and foreign particles. Little hairs called *cilia* beat back and forth to move the mucus and dirt up where it can be expelled by coughing or sneezing. There are other specialized cells in the airways called *macrophages*. Macrophages are cells that move around the body eating up toxins in the airways and lungs. There are two requirements for this system to work: (1) A regular supply of air containing oxygen must be inhaled through open, clear airways to reach the air sacs; and (2) the waste gas, carbon dioxide, must be exhaled through these same airways. A disruption in the normal functioning will result in diseases of the lung, as in the inflammatory process seen in a lupus patient.

Pleurisy can be complicated with *pneumonitis* (a type of pneumonia), making it difficult to differentiate between a lupus complication and an infection in the lungs. Pneumonitis can be acute (sudden) or chronic (long term). Patients may have such vague symptoms as shortness of breath, cough, and fever. An analysis of the pleural fluid can help differentiate between an infection of a bacterial or inflammatory origin. If there is a bacterial infection, treatment with antibiotic therapy is indicated. Fever is a symptom of acute pneumonitis and usually responds to corticosteroids or other immunosuppressive therapy.

In chronic pneumonitis, elasticity of the lungs declines over a long period leading to a condition known as *fibrosis*. The patient with fibrosis will experience progressive difficulty in breathing (*dyspnea*) and widespread infiltrates or fluid collection in the lungs. Immunosuppressive treatment is indicated for this uncommon but serious lung complication.

Another rare complication is pulmonary hemorrhage (bleeding in the lungs). Coughing up blood (*hemoptysis*) may be the first symptom of this condition and occurs in 11 percent of lupus patients. It is more common in young women. This lung complication is very serious and can result in death.

Pulmonary hypertension is another rare complication seen in some lupus patients. In this condition, pressure in the pulmonary artery (the blood vessel that leads from the heart to the lungs) rises above normal. The patient may experience shortness of breath upon minimal exertion, fatigue, chest pain, dizzy spells, and fainting. In the United States, an estimated 500 to 1,000 new cases of primary pulmonary hypertension are diagnosed each year. Children and adults of all ages can develop pulmonary hypertension, though the greatest number is reported in women between ages twenty and forty. Women tend to be more symptomatic than men. When pulmonary hypertension occurs in the absence of a known cause, it is referred to as *primary pulmonary hypertension*. There are likely many unknown causes of primary pulmonary hypertension. In secondary pulmonary hypertension, the cause for the increase in pressure is known. Common causes of secondary pulmonary hypertension are breathing disorders such as emphysema and bronchitis. In other cases, secondary pulmonary hypertension can be the result of inflammatory or collagen vascular diseases such as scleroderma, CREST syndrome (a connective tissue disorder that usually affects the skin, blood vessels and in severe cases the lungs, digestive tract, or heart), or systemic lupus.

The treatment for patients with pulmonary hypertension will depend on the combination of symptoms and any other disease that may be present. Some of the current treatments include anticoagulants (blood thinners), calcium channel blockers, digoxin, diuretics, inhaled oxygen, bosentan (brand name Tracleer®), epoprostenol (brand name Flolan®), and treprostinil (brand name Remodulin®).

Pulmonary embolism (a blood clot in the lungs) is usually seen in patients with antiphospholipid antibodies (see Chapter 3), but it can also occur in patients with pulmonary hypertension. The clot can originate in veins anywhere in the body and can be triggered by the compression of a vein (venostasis) hypercoagulability (increased thickening of the blood), and inflammation of the walls of the blood vessels. These three underlying conditions are known as the Virchow triad, and they are all known risk factors for deep vein thrombosis (DVT) and pulmonary embolism. Some studies suggest that every patient with a thrombus or clot in the upper leg or thigh will have a pulmonary embolism. Clots that form in the segment of the femoral vein behind the knee (the popliteal segment) are the cause of pulmonary embolism in more than 60 percent of cases. Fatal pulmonary embolism often results from clots that originate in the deep veins of the arm or shoulder or in the veins of the pelvis. Pulmonary embolism is one of the most life-threatening conditions encountered during pregnancy and is reported to be the the leading cause of maternal death in the United States.

Pulmonary embolism is an extremely serious condition and can be fatal if not treated immediately. Symptoms include shortness of breath, chest pain, painful breathing, chest wall tenderness, back pain, shoulder pain, upper abdominal pain, temporary loss of consciousness, coughing up blood, wheezing, irregular heartbeat, and discomfort in the chest area.

Many patients with pulmonary embolism do not show any symptoms initially and some patients may display unusual symptoms, but pulmonary embolism is an emergency and requires immediate treatment. Patients usually present with primary or isolated complaints of seizure, loss of consciousness, abdominal pain, high fever, coughing up mucus, adult-onset asthma, or hiccoughs. Patients may also have an abnormal rhythm of the heart, generalized internal bleeding, or other nonspecific symptoms.

Treatment for pulmonary embolism is anticoagulant (blood thinning) drugs such as heparin, warfarin, or other anticoagulation medications. If the patient is having difficulty breathing, oxygen may be administered.

Some patients recovering from a pulmonary embolism may experience a chronic swelling of the leg and may develop leg ulcers. Compression stockings can help prevent the swelling and should be used in most patients after a first episode of deep vein blood clot.

Lung complications can be diagnosed by a complete physical examination, history, and other studies that may include an angiography, chest X-ray, other radiologic studies, echocardiogram, and pulmonary function tests.

Lung infections are common complications in patients with weakened immune systems. Such patients are susceptible to bacterial, viral, or fungal infections. Treatments for these conditions are antibiotics, antifungal medication, and other agents.

Heart

Lupus can damage the heart as well. Some of the complications that may affect lupus patients include:

- *Pericarditis:* This is an inflammation of the sac that surrounds the heart. This is the most common of the heart-related lupus complications.
- *Atherosclerosis* or hardening of the arteries that supply blood to the heart muscle: People with lupus are at greater risk of developing plaque in the arteries that may lead to coronary heart disease, and with that, the risk of heart attack.
- *Heart valve disease:* Up to 30 percent of people with long-standing lupus may develop thickened heart valves. Damaged heart valves make the lupus patient more susceptible to infections (endocarditis), blood clots, or heart failure.
- *Myocarditis:* This is an inflammation of the heart muscle. Although a rare condition, it can lead to problems with the muscles of the heart causing the heart to beat irregularly— either too rapidly or too slowly.

• *Pericardial tamponade*: This is a collection of blood in the sac of the heart. It can result as a complication of pericarditis or myocarditis.
• *Congestive heart failure*: This is a combination of weakness, edema, and shortness of breath produced by the inability of the heart to maintain adequate blood flow to the body and the lungs.

To understand these complications more fully, let's review how the heart works (see Figure 6). The heart is not a large organ; it is about the size of a person's clenched fist and weighs 10–12 ounces. It is hollow, roughly conical in shape, with the narrow end pointed downward to the left and slightly forward. Its location in the chest cavity is just to the left of the midline, behind the sternum (center bone of the chest), and between the second and sixth left ribs.

Figure 6. Cross-section View of the Heart

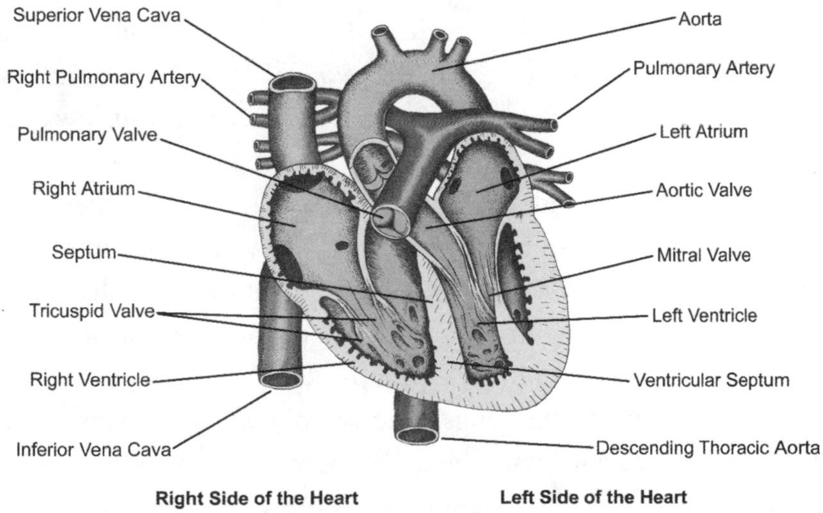

Left column labels: Superior Vena Cava, Right Pulmonary Artery, Pulmonary Valve, Right Atrium, Septum, Tricuspid Valve, Right Ventricle, Inferior Vena Cava

Right column labels: Aorta, Pulmonary Artery, Left Atrium, Aortic Valve, Mitral Valve, Left Ventricle, Ventricular Septum, Descending Thoracic Aorta

Right Side of the Heart   **Left Side of the Heart**

The wall of the heart consists of three layers:

- **Pericardium:** a fibrous sac surrounding the heart whose inner lining is a thin, transparent membrane covering the outside of the heart muscle
- **Endocardium:** the delicate innermost lining of the heart
- **Myocardium:** the thick muscular layer that separates the two linings.

The heart has four cavities, or chambers. Two of these are thin-walled receiving chambers—the left and right atria—and two are thick-walled pumping chambers—the ventricles.

Actually, the heart consists of two parallel pumps that work simultaneously. The right-sided pump receives deoxygenated blood (blood with no oxygen) from the veins and pumps it to the lungs where it is resupplied with oxygen. The left-sided pump receives the reoxygenated blood from the lungs and pumps it through the arteries to the rest of the body.

The heart contains four valves: the *tricuspid*, a valve between the right atrium and right ventricle; the *mitral* valve, between the left atrium and the left ventricle; the *pulmonic* valve, at the outflow area of the right ventricle; and the *aortic* valve, at the outflow area of the left ventricle.

The tricuspid and the mitral valves are open when the ventricles are filling and receiving blood from the atria but closed when the ventricles contract and are so structured that they prevent back-flow (regurgitation) of blood from the ventricle into the atrium. The right ventricle pumps blood into the pulmonary artery on its way to the lungs. The pulmonic valve opens when the ventricle contracts but closes during *diastole* (when the heart relaxes or rests after contraction), thus preventing the back-flow of blood from the pulmonary artery back into the right ventricle. The aortic valve opens when the left ventricle contracts to send blood into the aorta but closes during diastole so that blood cannot regurgitate from the aorta back into the left ventricle. The contraction of the ventricles and the closure of the valves contribute to the sounds of the heart.

Ventricular dysfunction is frequently seen in lupus patients. It results when the left ventricle of the heart is not working well (see Figure 6). The diagnosis of ventricular dysfunction is suspected when changes such as gallop rhythm (heartbeat that sounds like a galloping horse), a new heart murmur (abnormal sound of the heart), is detected in a physical examination. A chest X-ray may show an enlarged heart, and there may be abnormal changes in the electrocardiogram. An echocardiogram may also show abnormal functioning of the ventricle of the heart. (An echocardiogram is a sonogram where the physician can see how the heart moves and the size and shape of all the parts of the heart.)

The heart valves can become thickened in some lupus patients, a condition known as Libman-Sack vegetations or *verrucous endocarditis*. The *vegetations* are abnormal growths on the defective valves. This vegetation causes narrowing of the valves (stenosis), inability of the valves to close completely (regurgitation), or calcifications (calcium deposits), all which may require valve replacement. This condition affects the mitral valve most frequently, but the aortic and tricuspid valves may also be affected (see Figure 6). Patients are at risk of bacterial endocarditis with the presence of these vegetations. Bacterial endocarditis is diagnosed by a series of blood cultures in addition to the echocardiogram. In those patients with large vegetations, treatment consists of the use of anticoagulation therapy to decrease the formation of blood clots.

Arrhythmias, or abnormal heartbeats, occur in 10 percent of lupus patients. Sinus tachycardia (a nonthreatening increased rhythm of the heartbeat) is the most common type, found in up to 100 percent of the patients with active disease. It is diagnosed by an electrocardiogram. In the rare occasion when an abnormal rhythm becomes life threatening, a pacemaker can be used to regulate the heartbeat.

Coronary arteritis is a rare inflammation of the arteries of the heart. Patients with coronary arteritis may have angina (severe chest pain), heart attack, or both. Children and adults alike with lupus can be affected with this condition. The disease can be diagnosed by a series of coronary angiography (image of the heart artery in an X-ray taken after a special dye or substance has been injected into the patient's blood). It is important to distinguish between *arteritis* and *arteriosclerosis* because their treatments are quite different. Arteritis responds to corticosteroid therapy. In arteriosclerosis, surgery may be indicated.

Hypertension (high blood pressure) is a frequent complication in lupus. It often occurs in patients with kidney disease but can also be found in patients with arteriosclerosis. Hypertension is considered in those patients who on at least three occasions have a blood pressure of 140/90. (Under newer diagnostic guidelines issued the the Heart, Blood and Lung Institute, patients with 130/80 are considered to be at risk for hypertension.) Lupus patients with uncontrolled high blood pressure, with or without diabetes, may have an increased risk of heart attack. Treatment, depending on the patient's condition, consists of antihypertensive medication by itself or in conjunction with other medication and lifestyle changes.

As a result of early hardening of the arteries that can occur in both children and adults, lupus patients have a higher risk of coronary artery disease and heart attack (myocardial infarction). The presence of *anticardiolipin* antibodies (see Chapter 3: Immunologic Disorders) and the inflammation of the heart vessels can increase the risk of coronary artery disease (CAD). Physicians perform a coronary angiography to positively diagnose coronary artery disease. In an angiography, a very small tube or catheter is inserted into a blood vessel in the groin or arm. The physician guides the catheter through the blood vessel to the heart or at the beginning of the arteries supplying the heart, and a special dye—to provide contrast—is injected. This dye is visible on an X-ray, and the pictures that are obtained are called angiograms. Physicians can detect the degree of damage to the heart and vessels from the X-ray pictures. Another diagnostic tool is a specific sonogram study called an AB-mode sonogram. This sonogram can be used to determine early atherosclerotic changes. Various other studies are also available, and your doctor will decide which tests are right for you.

Treatment of coronary artery disease consists of lifestyle changes, such as dietary changes, adopting an exercise regimen, control of other diseases (like diabetes and hypertension) that increase the risk of heart attack, medications to lower the cholesterol level (if above 200), and other medications as required. Specific therapy will depend on the patient's condition.

GASTROINTESTINAL SYSTEM

Lupus patients may also experience gastrointestinal (GI) problems such as abdominal pain and diarrhea. Gastrointestinal problems can be caused by inflammation or damage to the small and large intestines, inflammation of the pancreas (pancreatitis), inflammation of the abdomen (peritonitis), enlargement of the spleen (splenomegaly), and enlargement of the liver (hepatomegaly).

The gastrointestinal tract (see Figure 7) performs the complex functions of digesting food and absorbing nutrients into the body while eliminating harmful substances. When this process breaks down, due to stresses caused by improper nutrition, toxins, emotional factors, illness, inadequate absorption of nutrients, or increased absorption of undesirable elements in the bowel, it can lead to abnormal responses of the immune system and inflammatory conditions.

Food allergies and sensitivities; toxic products from pesticides, herbicides, and processed foods; as well as stressful emotional factors play a large role in altering the normal

Figure 7. Anatomy of the Gastrointestinal System

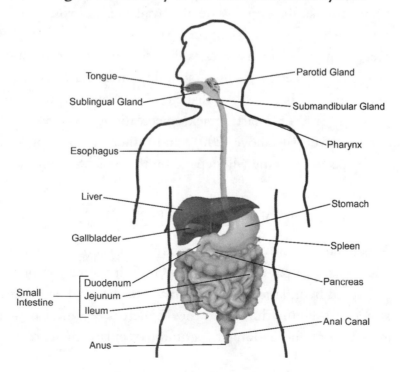

functioning of the gastrointestinal tract and the body's immune system. The result is a breakdown in the balance of the normal digestion and absorption processes and an abnormal permeability (leakiness) of the bowel. This condition, called "leaky bowel" syndrome, allows bacteria and ingested toxins to enter the blood stream. Some of these products are proteins called *antigens.* This infiltration of toxic particles can lead to some of the gastrointestinal problems lupus patients frequently encounter.

Thankfully, we can identify many of the factors that put the gastrointestinal function out of balance and consequently cause illness. Re-establishing the normal integrity of the bowel and the normal digestion and absorption processes is a very important first step in restoring the balance of the gastrointestinal tract. Physicians can perform a series of tests to determine the specific cause or the origin of the problem and prescribe appropriate treatmet.

Patients with complications of the stomach or *duodenum* (the beginning portion of the small intestine that starts at the end of the stomach) can develop ulcers, irritation, or inflammation of the stomach. Abdominal pain in the opening of the stomach is the most common symptom and may be relieved by eating some food or taking antacids. Patients with ulcers may develop nausea and vomiting. In some cases, bleeding or *perforation*, a hole or opening, can occur. The diagnosis of gastric or duodenal ulcers is made by a physical examination, an examination of the patient's medical history, an *endoscopy* (a procedure used to examine the interior of an organ) of the esophagus to the duodenum, or an upper gastrointestinal series (radiologic study). Treatment will depend on the findings of the studies.

Vasculitis is an inflammation in the *mesentery* (a sac in the abdomen that contains part of the intestine), the pancreas, the *peritoneum* (a sac that covers the entire abdomen), the liver, and the gall bladder. The inflammation may prevent normal blood flow or functioning of the affected organ. Vasculitis can result in abdominal pain, ulcers, bleeding, perforation, or even necrosis (death) of small segments of the intestine. Treatment will vary depending on the specific organs involved and may include intravenous fluids, antibiotics or other medications, and blood products. In extreme cases, surgery may be necessary.

Other problems involving the intestines may be thrombosis (formation of clots), especially in those patients with antiphospholipid antibodies (see Chapter 3), inflammatory bowel disease, drug-related disease (some medicines may contribute to ulcer formation), and fat malabsorption—the inability to properly digest fat products.

Pancreatitis (inflammation of the pancreas) can be present up to 23 percent of the time. It usually occurs in lupus patients with systemic multiple organ involvement. The patient may have severe abdominal pain that extends to the back, nausea, and vomiting. On rare occasions, pancreatitis may create a *fistula*. A fistula is an abnormal connection or bridge between organs or vessels that normally do not connect. *Pseudocysts* (abnormal sacs resembling cysts) may also form. Diagnosis of these conditions is made by analysis of the symptoms and blood work. Treatment includes intravenous fluids and pain medication. The patient may also be advised to avoid food intake in order to let the pancreas rest.

Lupus patients with liver disease can develop autoimmune hepatitis, a condition in which the patient's own immune system attacks the liver causing inflammation and liver cell death. It primarily affects women and can occur at any time during the course of the disease. The diagnosis is made when there is an increase in liver enzymes and there is no evidence of chronic hepatitis or other liver disease. Chronic hepatitis is the result of infections by viruses, toxins, drugs, or chemical abnormalities in the body. The types of viral hepatitis are commonly known as Hepatitis A, Hepatitis B, and Hepatitis C. These infections of the liver can be detected by a blood test called a hepatitis profile. Lupus patients with autoimmune hepatitis have a negative hepatitis profile but have a positive antibody test. Treatment is with immunosuppressive therapy.

KIDNEYS

As explained in Chapter 3, diseased kidneys may undergo a variety of changes as a result of the disease process. Hypertension is a persistent problem in lupus patients and is associated with lupus nephritis and increased risk for kidney failure and cardiovascular disease. Patients are treated with antihypertensive medication to prevent further damage to the kidneys. As part of the treatment, patients are advised to keep a diary of their blood pressure measurements, with instructions to contact medical personnel if their blood pressure increases or changes drastically from the recommended levels.

Nephrotic syndrome is another complication of kidney disease seen in lupus patients. In rare cases, it may be the presenting symptom, especially in children. Patients have *edema* (swelling due to water retention), *albuminuria* (increased levels of albumin, a blood protein, in the urine), decreased levels of albumin in the blood, and increased blood cholesterol. (Albumin is a major component of plasma proteins. It is influenced by nutritional state, the healthy functioning of the liver, kidneys, and various diseases such as nephrotic syndrome.) Nephrotic syndrome is treated with careful monitoring of fluids, corticosteroids, limitation of salt intake, diuretics, and other agents. Unresponsive or untreated nephrotic syndrome can result in several complications, such as renal (kidney) failure and hypertension. The increased levels of cholesterol seen in nephrotic syndrome can result in complications of the heart.

Thrombotic diathesis, an inherited predisposition to develop blood clots, can result from multiple risk factors in lupus patients. Two of these are nephrotic syndrome and the presence of antiphospholipid antibodies. These conditions alter the normal coagulation, or clotting of the blood, and can result in the formation of blood clots throughout the body. Treatment is anticoagulation (blood thinning) therapy as well as treatment of the underlying disease causing the production of the blood clots.

Chronic renal insufficiency (chronic kidney disease) results when the kidneys have not been functioning well for a prolonged period of time. Patients need to follow a low-protein diet, avoid salt and salt substitutes, as well as other restricted foods and substances, and supplement their diet with vitamin D. Chronic kidney disease should be treated aggressively as further or continued damage can result in kidney failure. Patients with kidney disease may experience nausea, vomiting, loss of appetite, anemia, lethargy, itching, and varying levels of consciousness depending on the severity of the condition and response to therapy. In children with lupus, high blood pressure with seizures may be the main symptoms of kidney failure or insufficiency. Some patients with kidney failure require long-term dialysis therapy. Dialysis is a procedure that filters metabolic waste products or toxins out of the blood through a catheter inserted into the vein (hemodialysis) or abdomen (peritoneal dialysis). Some patients can perform dialysis themselves after receiving adequate training and healthcare recommendations. The selection of which type of dialysis to follow depends greatly on the condition of the patient and the determinations made by the healthcare team.

If the kidneys have failed completely, some patients may need a kidney transplant. Kidney transplantation in lupus patients has been as successful as in non-lupus patients. The best time for a kidney transplant in a lupus patient is after a period of at least twelve months without any disease flare-up. Lupus activity can be followed by antibody measurements such as the double-stranded DNA test (see Chapter 3). In rare cases, kidney disease may also affect the transplanted kidney.[1]

MUSCULOSKELETAL SYSTEM

Lupus patients with arthritis can have several disease complications that affect their joints. The most frequently reported are the following:

Deformity

Deformity of the joints may develop without the bone changes seen in rheumatoid arthritis. This is most frequently observed in the joints of the hands. The "swan neck" deformity of the hand is one of the deformities encountered. This deformity involves the second and third finger of the hand—the thumb is considered the first finger.

Deformities of the hand can occur when ligaments become so stretched that they become lax or loose and can no longer return to normal, similar to an elastic band that has been stretched out too long and cannot return to its regular size or strength. In

---

1. In general, African-American patients have worse hypertension along with renal disease than European-American patients.

addition, tendons, bands that connect the muscle to the bone, may lose their stability and shift from side to side. This shifting is called *subluxation*. Both conditions can lead to joint imbalance as the bones are no longer being held firmly in place. Physical therapy and surgical correction of the affected structures are some of the treatments to be followed in these cases.

Joint effusion

Fluid that escapes from blood vessels or from the lymphatic system may be due to a joint infection known as *septic arthritis*. Symptoms that may be present with the joint swelling are increased pain and increased temperature of the affected joint. The doctor may perform a procedure known as a *joint tap*, in which a needle is inserted into the affected joint to extract fluid. The fluid, called *synovial* fluid, is located inside the joint area. The extracted fluid is sent to a laboratory to determine if a bacterial infection is producing the swelling. If this is the case, antibiotic therapy may be prescribed.

Pain

Persistent pain in the hip area may be a symptom of a condition known as *avascular necrosis* (AVN). Avascular necrosis is the result of insufficient blood supply to the affected area. This causes the tissues to die (necrosis). Some patients experience persistent pain of the hip joint as a side effect of long-term corticosteroid therapy. Some cases of persistent pain may be related to small blood vessel inflammation, (see Chapter 5) Raynaud's phenomenon (see Chapter 4) which can lead to vasospasm, the narrowing of the blood vessels described in Chapter 4, or antiphospholipid antibodies (explained in Chapter 3). *Fat emboli*

Figure 8. Human Skeleton

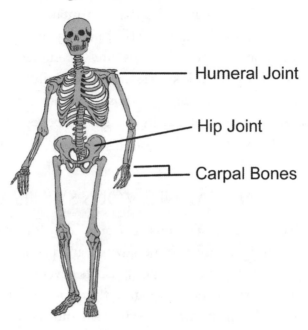

Humeral Joint

Hip Joint

Carpal Bones

may also cause pain. This is a condition similar to a blood clot, but instead of blood, the clot is formed from fat.

Avascular necrosis is commonly seen in the hips, carpal bones of the wrist, and the shoulders (see Figure 8). These bone changes are confirmed through X-rays or MRIs in addition to a clinical evaluation. Treatment will depend on the severity, location, and the degree of joint involvement. Treatment varies from observation to surgical correction in more severe cases.

Osteoporosis

Osteoporosis is another condition that the lupus patient may encounter as a side effect of prolonged corticosteroid therapy. Osteoporosis is usually reversible by adding supplemental calcium and vitamin D to the diet or by taking other prescribed medication. The recommended calcium intake is 1,500 mg per day and 800 international units (IUs) per day of vitamin D.

In addition, lifestyle changes are recommended, such as quitting smoking and drinking less alcohol. Daily weight-bearing exercises are recommended for those patients who are able to exercise. A bone mineral density test should be repeated every six months to follow the patient's improvement.

CENTRAL NERVOUS SYSTEM

Forty-five percent of lupus patients develop neurological complications in addition to the seizures and psychoses described in Chapter 3. In most cases lupus patients develop more than one neurological complication throughout the course of their disease. Headache is the most common symptom and is often the first to occur. Headaches in lupus tend to be the result of inflammation of the blood vessels (migraine or migraine related) or may be caused by tension. In most patients, headaches are harmless, but they occasionally occur as a result of complications of kidney disease, hypertension, or a reaction to corticosteroid therapy.

If a lupus patient suddenly begins to experience headaches that seem to have no other cause, he or she may have developed a condition known as *cerebritis*, which is an inflammation of the brain, or *cerebral venous thrombosis*, blood clots in the brain. Seizures can also be the result of inflammation of the brain vessels (lupus vasculitis), uncontrolled hypertension, blood clots, or bleeding. Some patients may have abnormalities of the cranial nerve (a nerve in the brain), vision disorders, or movement disorders such as *chorea* or Guillain-Barré syndrome. Chorea, also called St. Vitus Dance, is a disorder in which the patient makes involuntary movements of the face, limbs, or body. It is more common in children than in adults.

Strokes can occur in lupus patients with anticardiolipin antibodies (see Chapter 3), advanced hardening of the arteries, or inflammation of the blood vessels in the brain. In general, complications of the central nervous system respond to corticosteroid therapy and other immunosuppressive agents. (Please refer to Chapter 6 for further details on treatment.)

BLOOD DISORDERS

Multiple blood disorders, in addition to those discussed in Chapter 3, occur frequently in lupus patients. Anemia is the most common, affecting more than 50 percent of patients. It is the result of a decrease in red blood cell production.

Anemia may be due to the following factors:

- Inflammation secondary to disease activity
- Kidney-related decrease in the production of the hormone called *erythropoietin* that stimulates the bone marrow to produce red blood cells
- Decreased levels of iron
- Depression of the bone marrow as a result of medication.

Anemia results in a decrease of *hemoglobin*, the major protein of the red blood cells that helps transport oxygen from the lungs to the body. The normal range of hemoglobin levels in women is between 12.0 and 15.5; in men, between 13.6 and 17.5.

Patients with anemia may experience fatigue, faster than normal heartbeat (tachycardia), palpitations, dizziness, sensitivity to cold, paleness, weakness, headache, fatigue, or a general feeling of not being well. Treatment will depend on the cause; it may involve the use of corticosteroid therapy, iron supplements, or erythropoietin injections to stimulate the bone marrow to produce more red blood cells.

The first symptom of lupus in adults and children may be a decreased platelet count known as *idiopathic thrombocytopenia purpura* (ITP). This is a condition in which the number of platelets drop without any apparent cause, such as other disease or as a side effect of medication. It can become serious if left untreated.

Another rare complication of platelets in lupus patients is *thrombotic thrombocytopenic purpura* (TTP). In thrombotic thrombocytopenic purpura, patients will display symptoms of hemolytic anemia, thrombocytopenia, (rapid destruction of platelets faster than they can be replaced), fever, neurological symptoms, and kidney problems. Thrombotic thrombocytopenic purpura in lupus patients can be difficult to diagnose as the symptoms of active lupus can be almost identical to the ones seen in thrombotic thrombocytopenic purpura. Thrombotic thrombocytopenic purpura is a severe condition and can result in death if not treated. Luckily, the patient has a good chance of survival if given immediate plasma transfusions and a treatment process called *plasmapheresis* in which plasma is cleaned through a machine similar to that used with dialysis patients. In cases that do not respond to other therapies, the spleen may have to be removed.

Myelofibrosis, or the replacement of bone marrow with fibrous tissue, is a rare complication of thrombocytopenia. It may result from an abnormal transformation of red blood cells or anemia due to abnormalities or premature cells in the bone marrow. Thrombocytopenia can cause multiple complications in lupus patients. Treatment involves the use of immunosuppressive therapy.

Pure red blood cell aplasia is another type of anemia that can result from abnormal functioning of the bone marrow in its production of red blood cells. Patients are treated with immunosuppressive therapy, such as corticosteroids, and erythropoietin has also been used. In cases where the anemia is the result of an infection, and not due to lupus, gammaglobulin may be used for therapy. Gammaglobulin is a blood protein component containing multiple antibodies, thereby making it useful in protecting the immune system.

Thromboembolism is not common in lupus, but when it occurs it can result in serious complications. A blood clot, or thrombus, breaks off and travels through in the bloodstream forming the embolism. Blood clots may affect a number of places in the body, such as the veins of the legs where the blood clot forms, and can travel to the lungs, causing a pulmonary embolism. Clots can also form in the arteries that take blood to the arms, legs, or brain. During pregnancy, blood clots can lodge in the placenta and disrupt the supply of nutrients to the fetus. This can cause the baby to be born prematurely, with low birth weight, or even decrease its chances for survival. Repeated blood clot formation is a frequent complication in patients with anti-Ro and antiphospholipid antibodies. Treatment involves anticoagulation medication and other therapy to treat the underlying condition.

ENDOCRINE SYSTEM

Lupus patients can develop thyroid problems because of autoimmune problems not yet well understood. There are two types of thyroid diseases: *hyperthyroidism* and *hypothyroidism*. In hyperthyroidism, the thyroid is overactive, and the patient can develop osteoporosis, *myopathy* (muscular weakness), peri-arthritis (inflammation around the joint), or *acropachy* (clubbing of the fingers). Thyroid problems are more frequent in women.

In hypothyroidism, the thyroid is underactive. Patients with underactive thyroids may develop joint pains, arthritis, carpal tunnel syndrome, myopathy, a neuromuscular disease in which the muscle fibers do not function for a variety of reasons, or gout, a condition where the body produces excess uric acid that lodges in the joints. Most patients respond well to thyroid therapy, which may involve supplementation in the case of hypothyroidism, or suppression of the activity of the thyroid in the case of hyperthyroidism.

Diabetes can develop in lupus patients who have had long-term corticosteroid therapy. Corticosteroids cause an increase in blood sugar levels, which can lead to diabetes after prolonged use at high dosages. Diabetes can also be caused by some sort of autoimmune process.

As we have seen, the complications of lupus will vary from patient to patient depending on the stage of their disease and the presence or absence of other diseases or disorders that may worsen or exacerbate its symptoms. Additional complications may also occur and are not limited to the ones discussed in this chapter.

CHAPTER SIX

❧

TREATMENTS

SHAWNTINA'S STORY

I am only fourteen, but I've been diagnosed with lupus for over a year. I used to be ashamed of my condition, and I would try to hide it at school and from my friends. When I was first diagnosed, and before I started taking medication, I couldn't walk very well; I was shaky. My grades started to slip and I found myself wandering, even in biology—my favorite class. Some of the kids at school laughed at me and made fun of the way I walked, the slow way I got around. But, thanks to the support of my doctor and my family, I am no longer embarrassed. I tell people that I have lupus and I keep my head up high. My grades are up and my friends have become more supportive. Lupus can make anyone hysterical, especially when you are a teenager! But I wake up in the morning and thank God that I am alive. I sometimes feel like a walking miracle!

❧

Treatments for lupus depend on the form of lupus the patient has and whether or not there are any other diseases present. As emphasized, there are many kinds of treatment plans because there are many kinds of lupus patients. This chapter explains some of those treatments.

NONSTEROIDAL ANTI-INFLAMMATORY DRUGS

Nonsteroidal anti-inflammatory drugs are used for mild lupus symptoms. Some of these symptoms are fever, joint pain, and arthritis. Nonsteroidal anti-inflammatory drugs should be avoided in lupus patients with kidney disease because they can worsen kidney function. Also, ibuprofen should be avoided because it has been related to viral meningitis (inflammation of the membranes that protect the brain and nerves). Other common side effects of nonsteroidal anti-inflammatory drugs are distress of the gastrointestinal tract, including heartburn (reflux), gastric pain, gastric ulcer and bleeding, rash, dizziness, increased liver enzymes, fluid retention, allergic reaction, easy bruising, kidney toxicity, and blood changes.

Nonsteroidal anti-inflammatory drugs can inhibit the blood's ability to clot properly and may interact with blood-thinning medications, such as Coumadin®. Nonsteroidal anti-inflammatory drugs must be taken only upon the recommendation of a physician as they may interact negatively with other medications that the patient might be taking for other conditions. Also, patients need to take these medications with food. If unusual symptoms occur while taking the medication, notify your physician immediately. Dosage and drug selection will depend on each particular case.

Some nonsteroidal anti-inflammatory drugs, such as aspirin and ibuprofen, are available over the counter. Such preparations of ibuprofen include Aleve®, Motrin®, Advil®, Nuprin®, Midol®, Actron®, and others. Over-the-counter preparations of aspirin include Anacin®, Ascriptin®, Bayer® aspirin, Bufferin®, Alka-Seltzer®, Buffaprin®, Buffasal®, Ecotrin®, Empirin®, Excedrin®, Genprin®, Measurin®, ZORprin®, and others.

Other nonsteroidal anti-inflammatory drugs are available only by prescription. Below is a list of some of these (generic name first, brand name in parentheses):

- Diclofenac potassium (Cataflam®)
- Diclofenac sodium (Voltaren®)
- Diflunisal (Dolobid®)
- Fenoprofen (Nalfon®)
- Flurbiprofen (Ansaid®)
- Indomethacin (Indocin®)
- Ketoprofen (Orudis, Oruvail®)
- Meclofenamate sodium (Meclomen®)
- Meloxicam (Mobic®)
- Nabumetone (Relafen®)
- Naproxen (Naprosyn® and Naprelan®)
- Naproxen sodium (Anaprox®)
- Oxaprozin (Daypro®)
- Piroxicam (Feldene®)
- Sulindac (Clinoril®)
- Tolmetin sodium (Tolectin®)

There is a subclass of nonsteroidal anti-inflammatory drugs called cox-2 inhibitors. These include celecoxib (Celebrex®), rofecoxib (Vioxx®), and valdecoxib (Bextra®).

Doctors do not recommend combining nonsteroidal anti-inflammatory drugs because this increases the risk of potential side effects. Please check with your doctor before taking *any* pain-killer, over-the-counter medicines, or other prescription drugs.

ACETAMINOPHEN

Acetaminophen is often recommended to relieve mild joint pain, mild headaches, or fevers. It can be safely combined with anti-inflammatory medicines (nonsteroidal anti-inflammatory drugs), at the recommended dosage, because it does not cause stomach upset. It rarely causes allergies, rash, or blood changes. Care must be taken, however, not to exceed the recommended dose or take additional over-the-counter medications that contain acetaminophen. When taken in large doses, liver damage is possible. When alcohol or antipsychotic medications are taken together with acetaminophen, increased liver toxicity may result. Acetaminophen can increase the anticoagulant effect of warfarin, an oral anticoagulant.

Several commercial preparations are available over the counter, such as Panadol® and Tylenol®.

STEROIDS

Steroids or corticosteroids are frequently used to treat acute chronic lupus. Steroids are a hormone normally produced by the adrenal glands in small amounts, but in special cases, like lupus, commercial steroids are given to reduce inflammation and to suppress the activity of the overactive immune system. Steroids may be given to lupus patients by mouth (orally), injection, intravenous infusion (IV), or directly on the skin where needed. The most commonly prescribed oral steroid is prednisone.

Other oral corticosteroids are prednisolone, Medrol®, and dexamethasone. Methylprednisolone is given intravenously when a large dose of corticosteroids is needed. This is known as *pulse therapy* and is used in patients suffering from acute symptoms of lupus. Commercial preparations available are Solu-Medrol®, Solu-Cortef®, and Decadron®. Caution should be taken in patients with diabetes, atherosclerosis, hypertension, osteoporosis, infections, peptic ulcer, and cirrhosis because steroids can cause complication in these diseases. Topical steroids can be used to treat the skin rashes. They need to be used cautiously and only as needed, because sun exposure can cause topical steroids to alter and irritate the skin. Preparations are available in ointments or creams.

Most of the side effects of corticosteroids are dose related. Side effects are more frequently encountered when high doses are taken for more than a few weeks. Side effects may include facial puffiness, weight gain, increased appetite, bruising, edema (fluid retention), high blood pressure, osteoporosis, decreased calcium levels in the body, diabetes, stretch marks, acne, cataract, insomnia, mood changes, personality change, psychosis, arteriosclerosis, muscle weakness, fractures, and increased susceptibility to infections. **Steroids must never be stopped abruptly.**[2]

CALCIUM AND VITAMIN D

Calcium and vitamin D supplementation are recommended for lupus patients undergoing corticosteroid therapy in order to prevent or improve any bone changes. Side effects may include hypercalcemia (elevated calcium levels), hypercalciuria (excretion of high levels of calcium in the urine), and kidney stones. Caution

---

2. PATIENT ADVISORY: Do not attempt to stop steroid treatment on your own without your doctor's knowledge and authorization. Doing so can be very dangerous, possibly fatal. When taken in large doses and/or for a prolonged period, this medication needs to be reduced gradually.

should be taken when used in conjunction with a diuretic called thiazide, because it can abnormally increase the calcium levels in the blood. Over-the-counter preparations are available, including Calciferol (ergocalciferol, a form of vitamin D2) and Rocaltrol (calcitriol, a form of vitamin D).

HYDROXYCHLOROQUINE (PLAQUENIL®)

Hydroxychloroquine (Plaquenil®) is an anti-malarial drug used frequently in mild disease, especially in the treatment of skin and joint problems. Another anti-malarial preparation often prescribed is chloroquine (Aralen®). Both are administered orally. Because there is a risk of retinal damage and blurry vision with these medications, patients are directed to have their eyes examined by an ophthalmologist before starting anti-malarial therapy and every six months thereafter.

Other side effects may include the following:

- Irritation to the gastrointestinal tract
- Headaches and emotional changes
- Skin rash, itchiness, and blue/black coloration of the skin (rare)
- Liver and kidney problems
- Ototoxicities (damage to the ears) (rare)
- Reversible corneal opacities, irreversible retinal damage (rare)
- Blood dyscrasias (imbalances) or hemolysis (breakdown of red blood vessels with G6PD (Glucose-6–phosphate dehydrogenase) deficiency.

Caution should be taken in patients with liver diseases, psoriasis, and *porphyria*, a group of blood-related disorders affecting the skin and the nervous system.

CHEMOTHERAPEUTIC DRUGS

Chemotherapeutic drugs are often used to help control moderate to severe lupus with organ involvement. They are also used in vasculitis, rheumatoid arthritis, polymyositis (inflammation of the muscle fibers), or dermatomyositis (a disease characterized by skin rash and progressive muscle weakness).

Chemotherapeutic drugs, like steroids, suppress the immune system and have anti-inflammatory effects. Close monitoring is indicated in all of them. Patients need to follow the therapy as prescribed and should report any bleeding, fever, or other unusual symptoms to their physicians. This class of drugs includes cyclophosphamide (Cytoxan®), methotrexate (Folex®, Rheumatrex®), and azathioprine (Imuran®). While using these drugs, patients should avoid any live virus vaccines.

Cyclophosphamide

Use of this drug requires frequent monitoring with a complete blood count and platelet counts. White blood counts usually decrease after 7–14 days of this treatment, so this measurement is used to help monitor the dose to be used in the next treatment. Also, a urine test is used to monitor for blood in the urine with long-term use of the medication. Side effects will vary depending on the dose and length of time the drug is used and may include the following:

- Gastrointestinal problems (vomiting, diarrhea, and nausea)
- Hair loss
- Increased risk of infections (usually bacterial and viral infections with opportunistic [rare] organism)
- Permanent infertility
- Bladder bleeding (hemorrhagic cystitis)
- Suppression of bone marrow

- Pulmonary fibrosis
- Rash
- Hypersensitivity reaction
- Risk of developing a malignancy, including bladder cancer, lymphoma, leukemia, and skin cancers, with some cases of long-term use.

Caution should be taken when using allopurinol because it increases the bone marrow suppression of Cytoxan®. Leukopenia may be prolonged with the used of thiazide diuretics. Cytoxan® may decrease the therapeutic levels of digoxin (a heart medication).

Methotrexate

This medication is should not be given to patients with allergic reaction to the drug's components, or those with liver disease, kidney dysfunction, alcoholism, or during pregnancy. Alcohol or any over-the-counter medication that contains alcohol should be avoided because it may result in liver damage. Side effects include gastrointestinal upset, malaise, temporary elevation of liver enzymes, mucositis (which can develop to oral ulcers), and, in some cases, lung toxicity.

Azathioprine

This medication is contraindicated (not recommended) in cases of hypersensitivity, when taking allopurinol, and during lactation or pregnancy. Side effects include fever, chills, vomiting, diarrhea, nausea, and depending on the dose, bone marrow suppression.

Mycophenolate (Cell Cept®)

This is an immunosuppressive drug used for the treatment of certain types of lupus nephritis and to prevent organ transplant rejection. Side effects include sensitivity to infections, diarrhea, constipation, stomach pain, upset stomach, vomiting, difficulty falling asleep or staying asleep, decreased platelet counts, and pain in the back, muscles, or joints. Rare side effects include swelling of the hands, feet, ankles, or lower legs; difficulty breathing; difficulty shaking hands; unusual bruising or bleeding; headaches; fast heartbeat; excessive tiredness; dizziness; pale skin; weakness; bloody or "coffee grounds" vomiting; black and tarry stools; red blood in stools; and loose and watery stools. Mycophenolate needs to be supervised closely via frequent blood tests.

FOLIC ACID

This is a vitamin used to decrease the side effects of methotrexate. It is usually taken once a day. One brand preparation is called Folvite®. Adverse effects are rare but may include a rash or flushing of the skin. It is contraindicated for patients with vitamin B12 deficiency.

MESNA

This is a drug used to prevent hemorrhagic cystitis (bleeding from the bladder) when using cyclophosphamide or ifosfamide therapy. The brand name is Mesnex®. Side effects may include bad taste in the mouth, headache, diarrhea, nausea, musculoskeletal pain, hives, and allergic rash.

EYE DROPS

Lubricating eye drops are indicated for dry eyes. There are many commercial preparations available over the counter and by prescription. The regular use of preservative-free solutions will help prevent irritation of the eyes, but they can also cause blurry vision. Sanitary precautions, such as washing one's hands prior to using the drops and preventing the dropper from contacting the eye, are generally advised.

CALCITONIN

Calcitonin is a hormone used for the treatment and prevention of osteoporosis. Several commercial brands are available in an injectable form or as a nasal spray. Injectable versions include Calcimar® (salmon calcitonin) and Cibacalcin® (human calcitonin); Miacalcin® (salmon preparation) is a nasal spray. Some side effects that can occur with calcitonin use include headaches, flushing, nausea, diarrhea, injection-site reaction, chills, tingling sensation, rash, hypersensitivity, rhinitis (irritation or inflammation in the nose), and nasal irritation.

CALCIUM SALTS

Calcium supplements are used for the treatment of osteoporosis or hypocalcemia. Numerous over-the-counter calcium products are available. Some of these are Citracal®, Neo-Calglucon®, Alka-Mints®, Caltrate®, Os-cal®, Oyst-Cal®, Calci-Chew®, Rolaids Calcium Rich®, Titralac®, Tums®, Tums E-X®, and Viactiv®. Calcium supplements should be taken with a large glass of water with a meal and should not be taken within one to two hours of another medication. Do not take calcium if you have kidney stones, hypercalcemia (increased calcium levels in the blood), digoxin toxicity, or kidney failure. Possible side effects of these supplements include constipation, flatulence, nausea, kidney stones, and hypercalcemia.

CAPSAICIN

Capsaicin is a topical analgesic used for the relief of joint or muscle pains. Several commercial solutions are available, including Zostrix®, Capsin®, Theragen®, Capsagel®, and Dolorac®. When applied to the skin, capsaicin can cause a temporary burning sensation in the area. In some cases, a rash may develop in the area of application.

CYCLOSPORINE

An immunosuppressive drug, cyclosporine is used in lupus and other rheumatologic conditions to decrease inflammation. Sandimmune® and Neoral™ are the two most widely used cyclosporine drugs. Cyclosporine should be avoided in patients with a history of malignancy, uncontrolled hypertension, or kidney or liver dysfunction. When on cyclosporine treatment, patients should avoid sunlight (to prevent skin cancer), and regular blood monitoring is important. Though dependent on the dosage used, side effects include hypertension, increased creatinine, hirsutism (unusual hair growth), nausea, cramps, tremor, gingival hypertrophy (abnormal enlargement or overgrowth of the gums), hyperkalemia (increased potassium levels), hypomagnesemia (increased magnesium levels), hyperuricemia (high levels of uric acid in the blood), seizures, headache, muscle cramps, allergy, myositis (swelling of the muscles), pancreatitis (inflammation of the pancreas), sensitivity to infections, and risk of malignancy (lymphoma).

ALENDRONATE

Alendronate, a bisphosphonate (medication to strengthen the bone) used to treat and prevent osteoporosis, is best known by the brand name Fosamax™. This drug is not recommended for patients with severe kidney insufficiency, hypersensitivity to drug components, hypocalcemia (low blood calcium), or esophageal dysmotility where the contractions in the esophagus become irregular, unsynchronized, or absent altogether. Headaches, nausea, dyspepsia, dysphagia (difficulty swallowing), rash, or irritation to the esophagus are all possible side effects of alendronate.

AMITRYPTYLINE HYDROCHLORIDE

This is an antidepressant drug known commercially as Elavil® or Endep®. It is used for depression, insomnia, and fibromyalgia (an arthritis-like condition characterized by generalized muscular pain and fatigue); however, it is also used to help control chronic pain and migraines. Patients recovering from a heart attack, with irregular heartbeats, or with glaucoma are generally ill-advised to take amitryptyline. Patients with a history of hyperthyroidism, kidney, or liver problems must be cautious in taking this drug and be alert to unusual physical responses. If the medication is taken in large doses, it should not be discontinued suddenly. Tolerance, or reduced drug effectiveness, often occurs with continued use. Patients should avoid alcohol when taking amitryptyline. Side effects can include sedation, blurry vision, dry eyes, dry mouth, drowsiness, constipation, difficulty with urination, postural hypotension, restlessness, tremor, Parkinsonian syndrome (symptoms similar to Parkinson's disease), liver damage, alopecia (hair loss), arrhythmias (irregular heartbeat), breast enlargement, and blood changes.

PLASMAPHERESIS

Plasmapheresis is a procedure indicated for patients who have lupus nephritis or hemolytic anemia with a rapidly deteriorating course. In this procedure, plasma proteins such as immunoglobulins (antibody proteins) are removed from the blood to help to improve immune system function. Most often used in conjunction with cyclophosphamide, plasmapheresis removes the proteins that react against the patient's own cells to fight disease. It is a controversial procedure because it is expensive and high risk.

BLOOD TRANSFUSION

In some cases, blood transfusions may be recommended to treat an acute complication of lupus. There are a variety blood products that can be used during a transfusion, including red blood cells, platelets, plasma, serum, or whole blood; the type of transfusion needed will depend on the specific disorder present at that time.

Everyone is concerned about the possibility of infections during blood transfusions. Fortunately, blood screening has become extremely effective. The current risk of contracting human immunodeficiency virus (HIV) and hepatitis from a blood transfusion today is very low because all blood products are thoroughly screened, and any units that test positive for disease are discarded. But while blood testing is better today, the process remains imperfect, which is why additional information is requested from prospective blood donors. The additional questioning about the donor's medical and social history has helped improve the screening process. If any information is suspicious or if risk factors for diseases are detected, the blood is not used.

However, because blood transfusions are not absolutely safe, transfusion is reserved for times when the alternate risk of not transfusing would be significant. In case of an elective surgery, the doctor may advise the patient to set aside his or her own blood for possible transfusion. Such blood is referred to as *autologous*. In addition, blood can also be donated by friends or relatives if the blood type is compatible. However, because one's closest friends and relatives may be reluctant to reveal personal lifestyle information that affects how safe they are as donors, their blood is not necessarily safer than blood from a blood bank.

NEW THERAPIES

There are several medications that are being evaluated for their effectiveness in treating lupus and related conditions:

- *Hormone therapy:* In patients with lupus, a necessary natural hormone, *dehydroepiandrosterone* (DHEA) is very low. There is some evidence that dehydroepiandrosterone may alleviate some symptoms for lupus patients whose lupus affects only their skin and joints and may even reduce the need for other medication, but many other studies are required to understand the mechanism and benefits of this therapy before it can be widely prescribed.
- *Biological agents:* These drugs are relatively new and are used frequently in arthritis and other immunologic diseases. Their uses and benefits in lupus are not well understood and are still under investigation. Based in

compounds that occur naturally in our body, these agents selectively block parts of the immune system. Some of the biologics under investigation are Enbrel®, Remicade®, and Humira®.

- *Stem cell transplantation:* Stem cell transplantation has been successful in some studies. Stem cells are harvested from the patient from blood or bone marrow and reserved. The patient then undergoes massive doses of chemotherapy to remove all traces of the original immune system. The stem cells are then reintroduced into the patient to restore the immune system to its state before the disease.

- *Belimumab:* This monoclonal antibody experimental drug inhibits the development of B-lymphocytes (a type of white blood cells) to prevent lupus flare-ups by restoring the normal process of cell death (apoptosis).

- *Mycophenolate mofetil (MMF):* This drug is under investigation to evaluate the efficacy and tolerability for the treatment of lupus nephritis in comparison to the present immunosuppressive therapies.

- *Rituximab (Rituxan®):* This is an immunosuppressive therapy that consists of a monoclonal antibody directed against CD20 cells. The drug is being evaluated in patients with moderate to severe lupus due to severe side effects that may develop with its use.

- *LJP 394:* This experimental drug is under evaluation for the prevention of kidney flare-ups.

- *Abatacept:* This drug is under evaluation for its effectiveness in preventing lupus flare-ups, especially for those patients with lupus involvement in at least three organ systems such as the skin, heart, and lungs, or arthritis in more than four joints.

• *MEDI-545:* This is a human monoclonal antibody given by intravenous infusion. This drug is being tested to evaluate its effectiveness in preventing lupus flare-ups by inhibiting interferon alpha subtypes, the agents that cause inflammation in lupus.

Lupus patients on drug therapies are usually carefully monitored with blood work and physical evaluation so that any complications that develop can be caught early. It is the patient's—or in the case of children, the caretaker's—responsibility to follow the doctor's instructions and not to alter or cease treatment without talking to the doctor first. Sudden discontinuation of some of medications can cause serious damage, and even death. Also, the patient must not take medications that have not been authorized by the physician, because certain drugs may interfere with the prescribed therapy. Furthermore, alternative therapies such as herbs, acupuncture, and nutritional supplements may also interfere with lupus treatment. If in doubt, it is best to check with the doctor or other healthcare practitioner before taking any kind of supplement.

CHAPTER EIGHT

>

PREGNANCY AND LUPUS

OVER A CENTURY AGO, pregnancy was not recommended for lupus patients, but improved treatments have made it possible for successful pregnancies to occur most of the time. However, since miscarriages continue to occur approximately 25 percent of the time, lupus patients are advised to seek medical and emotional counseling before becoming pregnant. The doctor will determine if the patient's health will permit a pregnancy, and the counselor will explore whether the patient is ready to take on the additional responsibilities of caring for a baby. All the risks must be understood prior to making the decision to become pregnant.

Because many problems can develop during a lupus pregnancy, it is considered to be high risk. An obstetrician and a rheumatologist generally stay quite involved in a lupus pregnancy. After medical and psychological professionals have approved a pregnancy, a great deal of planning around the patient's disease state is necessary. The best time to become pregnant is when the disease is in remission. This is usually when the treatment regimen has been stabilized and thus can be continued throughout the entire pregnancy. This is important because some medications, like the chemotherapeutic agents that are used to control organ involvement, cannot be used during pregnancy. In fact, pregnancy is discouraged in patients receiving chemotherapy because the medication can increase the risk of birth defects. Medications such as prednisone and methylprednisolone do not come in contact with the baby, so ordinarily they do not alter plans for pregnancy. However, if a woman becomes pregnant during an active, uncontrolled disease state, there can be serious complications.

If a lupus patient wishes to prevent pregnancy using a contraceptive, certain methods, such as intrauterine devices (IUDs), are not recommended because of the increased risk of infection. Other contraceptive devices that should be used with caution include the diaphragm and intrauterine substances or sponges. In addition, the use of oral contraceptives is not recommended for patients with a history of blood clots.

During pregnancy, the body undergoes several changes that a lupus patient may have difficulty adapting to, including a possible flare-up of the disease. The large increase in the amount of body fluid (about 30%) may be difficult for a lupus patient to tolerate, especially if she has kidney, cardiac, or vascular problems. There are also changes in the immune system and hormones during pregnancy, which can cause disease flare-ups. Possible symptoms the patient may experience are the following:

- Morning stiffness
- Fever
- Activation of the skin rash
- Stomach discomfort
- Joint pains

- Arthritis
- Fatigue
- Headaches
- Dizziness.

In general, pregnant women need to be carefully monitored during pregnancy to detect any signs of flare-up so treatment can be given early if necessary. Mild lupus flare-ups can usually controlled with prompt treatment, but further treatment can be administered depending on the patient's symptoms or if complications develop.

Several complications can occur during pregnancy that are unrelated to lupus. Hypertension (high blood pressure) can present in different ways during pregnancy. High blood pressure induced by pregnancy is defined as 140/90 and usually returns to normal after completion of the pregnancy. The patient may also have had hypertension before becoming pregnant. This results in *coincidental hypertension*, which is chronic hypertension in existence before the pregnancy and continuing after completion of the pregnancy. Chronic hypertension is considered one of the most common complications of pregnancy.

Some pregnant patients may have an increase in blood pressure late in the pregnancy, proteins in the urine, increased proteins in the blood, and mild edema. This condition is known as *toxemia* or *preeclampsia* and is more common in African-American women, older patients, women who are pregnant with twins, patients with kidney disease, and patients who smoke. In cases of preeclampsia, the platelet count can severely decrease. In the advanced stage of preeclampsia, patients may appear ill and develop complications of other organs, such as liver *infarcts* (death of tissue as a result of obstruction of blood supply), or congestive heart failure. Some of these symptoms can be confused with a lupus flare-up. Preeclampsia needs to be treated immediately to prevent serious complications including possible death to the mother and baby. Treatment may include antihypertensive medication, sedatives, or immediate delivery of the baby by cesarean section to decrease the stress of the mother.

Elevated blood pressure can also result in preeclampsia and eclampsia during pregnancy. In preeclampsia, the blood pressure can be 140/90 or higher and be accompanied in various combinations by proteinuria, headaches, pain in the upper middle part of the abdomen, and edema, or swelling of the face and hands.

Eclampsia is a serious complication of pregnancy and usually occurs after the onset of preeclampsia, although sometimes no preeclamptic symptoms are recognizable before its onset. The sypmptoms of eclampsia are similar to those in preeclampsia, but in eclampsia, convulsions or seizures are likely to occur.

HELLP syndrome can also occur during pregnancy. The acronym *HELLP* stands for the presence of *h*emolysis, *e*levated *l*iver enzymes, and *l*ow *p*latelets. This complication also occurs late in the pregnancy. Patients will develop fever, liver pain, and *encephalopathy* (disease of the brain). They are very ill, and there is a high risk of death for the baby and mother. This condition usually continues for several weeks after delivery.

Blood disorders can also occur during pregnancy. A possible combination of disorders is thrombocytopenia with anemia. Both usually resolve after pregnancy without complications. Another blood disorder is the increase in clotting factors. This can occur in clotting complications in patients with the antiphospholipid antibody (see Chapter 3). These changes are difficult to differentiate from a lupus flare-up during pregnancy. Other symptoms that may be present in a lupus flare-up and not in regular pregnancy are lupus rash, arthritis, and some types of neurological complications.

Heart disease occurs in one percent of pregnancies; they are usually related to congenital heart problems, defects of the heart valves, or pulmonary hypertension. Prognosis will depend on the patient's specific heart problem and response to therapy. Diabetes during pregnancy can be a preexisting condition or can develop secondary to pregnancy complications. This disease is usually treated with insulin and diet. Gestational diabetes can develop during pregnancy and occur late in the term. Risk factors include the following: the woman is at least thirty years of age, has a history of large babies in previous pregnancies, is obese, is hypertensive, and has increased glucose levels in the urine.

Some pregnant lupus patients, who may or may not be taking steroids, develop diabetes, pregnancy-induced hypertension, hyperglycemia (increased blood sugar), and kidney complications. The baby can have several complications during and after delivery, including chemical imbalance, decreased blood glucose, and developmental abnormalities. In general, pregnant women with lupus need to be monitored closely during the pregnancy in order to detect any complications so that adequate therapy can be administered as needed.

Another problem that can occur in lupus pregnancies is that the placenta, a temporary organ that supplies nutrients to the fetus, is sometimes small. This condition often occurs in patients with antiphospholipid antibodies, which can cause blood clots and lead to small areas of dead tissue in the placenta. The presence of antiphospholipid antibodies is associated with an increased risk of miscarriage. In fact, fetal loss can occur in up to 20 percent of pregnancies of mothers with antiphospholipid antibodies, especially in the presence of lupus anticoagulant and the IgG anticardiolipin antibodies. These episodes of fetal loss usually occur late in the first or second trimester of pregnancy. If these antibodies are detected early in the pregnancy, they may be treated with baby aspirin or heparin throughout the rest of the pregnancy to help to prevent miscarriages.

Antiphospholipid antibodies may cause blood clots in the placenta and therefore create several complications for the developing fetus. In addition, antiphospholipid antibodies are associated with other complications in pregnancy as well. These include separation of the placenta from the wall of the uterus, a condition known as *placental abruption*; an insufficient supply of blood to the placenta, leading to retardation of growth in the fetus; preeclampsia; and preterm birth. Preterm babies born to mothers with antiphospholipid antibodies may also have ventricular hemorrhage, and respiratory distress syndrome, that may require assisted ventilation in some cases. In spite of these problems, however, the good news is that most infants of mothers with antiphospholipid antibodies will not have any neurological or developmental abnormalities and will grow normally.

Usually, babies born to mothers with lupus do not have birth defects. However, roughly 25 percent of babies born to mothers with lupus are born prematurely. Furthermore, about 3 percent of babies born from lupus patients will have neonatal lupus. Though this condition goes away within a few months after birth, usually after the mother's antibodies are resolved and the baby has developed its own mature red blood cells, the baby is born with anti-Ro and anti-La antibodies. Babies with neonatal lupus may have skin rash, temporary abnormalities in the blood count, and a heart beat abnormality called "heart block."

The neonatal rash can take many forms but is usually scattered over the body and sometimes on the face. It appears a few days or weeks after birth, particularly after sun exposure, and usually disappears after a few weeks, leaving no scar. The rash often appears as a well-demarcated reddened, doughnut-shaped, scaly plaque predominantly on the scalp, neck, or face. This plaque typically occurs around the eyes, but similar plaques may also appear on the trunk. They are sometimes crusted and occur more often in male babies than in female babies.

Abnormal blood count conditions typically seen in neonatal lupus are low platelets, anemia, and other abnormalities. Seldom serious, these abnormalities usually go away in a few weeks without treatment. Heart block, an abnormal function of the heart that can be measured by an electrocardiogram can also occur. Though rare, damage from heart block is permanent. The normal heartbeat starts in the upper heart (the atria or auricles) and travels smoothly through to the bottom of the heart (the ventricles). In heart block, the atrial beat (normally about 140 times per minute in a newborn) cannot get through to the ventricles because scar tissue blocks its path. The ventricles then independently send the beats that determine the pulse (about 60 times per minute in a newborn), resulting in an abnormally slow pulse for a newborn.

Congenital heart block can often be diagnosed between the fifteenth and twenty-fifth week (fourth to sixth month) of pregnancy. If the fetus has heart block but appears to be doing well, either nothing is done or, in some cases, a special form of cortisone is given that will go through the placenta to the baby; however, cortisone may not make the heart beat normally again. If the baby is not doing well and is big enough to deliver, usually at thirty weeks into the pregnancy or later, delivery is often the best way of handling the problem. After birth, many babies with congenital heart block can live normal lives with no treatment, but some may need a pacemaker, and a small number may die from heart disease.

Neonatal lupus can also occur in babies of nonlupus mothers who have the anti-Ro antibodies in their blood. In such cases, babies will develop and grow normally if there are no other birth defects or congenital diseases. This is true for babies born from mothers with or without lupus.

A woman who has already had one child with neonatal lupus has about a 25 percent risk that her next child will develop the illness. Many women who deliver children with neonatal lupus do not have symptoms of lupus. In fact, except for their abnormal blood tests, many are well. Essentially, the specific characteristics (except for the antibodies) of the mother's diagnosis changes the risk of neonatal lupus. Lupus patients who are sick are no more or less likely to have a child with neonatal lupus than lupus patients who are well.

During the first two months after delivery there is an increased risk of lupus flare-ups in some patients. A frequent question asked by all lupus mothers is whether or not they are able to breast-feed their babies. This depends on the medications they are taking. Some medicines used to treat lupus will pass through the maternal milk and may be harmful to the baby.

PART III

RESEARCH AND RESOURCES

CHAPTER EIGHT

⌘

SOME POSSIBLE CAUSES

E TIOLOGY IS THE WORD doctors use to describe the science that deals with the cause or origin of disease and the factors that make one person more likely to develop a particular disease or condition. Unfortunately, in the case of lupus, the cause is still unknown despite intensive research. We do know, however, that certain genetic factors may be significant, and environmental factors are also being explored.

Genetic studies show that in identical twins with lupus the disease may be present in both twins up to 69 percent of the time in comparison to 5 percent of the time with nonidentical twins. This suggests that environmental factors and infectious and noninfectious agents may trigger lupus in individuals with a genetic predisposition to the disease.

ELSIE'S STORY

I was diagnosed with lupus in 1991, six months after the birth of my daughter, Liz. Ever since, my life has completely changed. Every time I was exposed to the sun, my skin would break out in a rash. In hot weather, I felt an incredible burning sensation inside my veins; I suffered from extreme fatigue. I live in Puerto Rico, where the weather is almost always hot—summer became my worst nightmare. I couldn't enjoy our famous beaches! But all is not lost, because even though I can't go the beach, I've created my own summer retreat at home, which I enjoy tremendously. I have shade trees, awnings, wind chimes, and an aboveground pool. I go outside to swim at dusk. And I don't have to get sand all over me!

I want everyone to know that it doesn't matter if you have lupus because you can live a normal life. Despite all of the changes in my life, I still have hope—and there are a lot of wonderful people out there making a tremendous effort to help. I've been through many stages of lupus, and right now I'm in remission. That means that my lupus is "asleep," or inactive, and I'm not planning to let it "wake up." I follow my doctor's instructions to the letter and take my medication religiously. I try to smile even on my worst days. I used to fight it all the time, but I've learned coping strategies to help me fight depression. I have found that smiling at life and keeping the faith has kept me strong.

Noninfectious factors include the following:

- *Sunlight:* Exposure to the ultraviolet light of the sun can activate the skin rashes of lupus (malar rash and discoid rash) and may also reactivate the systemic symptoms of lupus. One theory suggests that ultraviolet light causes certain cell proteins to accumulate on the surface of the cells, and these proteins then react with autoantibodies present in lupus patients. The result is a local or systemic inflammatory process. For this reason, we have emphasized that patients must avoid direct sun exposure, wear protective clothing (long pants, long shirt sleeves, hat), and use sunblock at all times while outdoors.

- *Stress:* Stress is thought to contribute to lupus flare-ups. Traumatic events such as death in the family, divorce, severe illness of a loved one, loss of job, and other life changes raise the levels of certain hormones in the body. Studies are underway to determine if these stress hormones influence or interfere with the course of the disease.

- *Chemical substances:* Certain medications have been linked to drug-induced lupus, or lupus-like syndrome. This syndrome has been reported more frequently in men than in women because men are more often treated with medications that result in this syndrome.

Lupus symptoms may develop after only months or years of using a drug, and they may resolve, or go away, when the drug is discontinued. Though symptoms and blood test abnormalities will disappear after a few months, an antinuclear antibody test may remain positive for several years.

A variety of symptoms are produced by drug-induced lupus: joint pains, arthritis, muscle pain, rash, swelling of the lymph nodes, pleurisy, pleural effusion, pericarditis, enlarged liver or spleen, kidney diseases, neurologic involvement, anemia, and low level of circulating white blood cells. Blood tests may also show such changes as elevated erythrocyte sedimentation rate (measures inflammation), Coombs positive (test for hemolysis, the breakdown of red blood cells), hypocomplementemia (missing blood complements), positive antinuclear antibody, rheumatoid factor, and production of antibodies to histones (a DNA protein), double-stranded DNA, and anti-Smith (see Chapter 3).

There are no specific criteria for the diagnosis of lupus-like syndrome because patients may have a variety of clinical and laboratory changes. Diagnosis is achieved by taking a detailed history, a physical examination, and confirming suspected etiology by blood tests. The diagnostic process is complex because symptoms are not specific and vary tremendously from person to person. Discontinuation of the offending substance is usually standard practice.

The drugs known to cause drug-induced lupus include the following:

- Chlorpromazine (antipsychotic)
- Hydralazine and methyldopa (for hypertension)
- Isoniazid (for tuberculosis)
- Minocycline (antibiotic)
- Procainamide and quinidine (for abnormal heartbeats).

A large number of other drugs may be associated with drug-induced lupus. Among anticonvulsive medications, these include the following:

- Benzodiazepines
- Carbamazepine
- Ethosuximide
- Hydantoin
- Phenytoin
- Primidone
- Trimethadione
- Valproate.

Among beta-blockers, medications that may be associated with drug-induced lupus are the following:

- Acebutolol
- Atenolol
- Labetalol
- Metoprolol
- Oxprenolol
- Pndolol
- Practolol
- Propranolol.

There are additional drugs associated with drug-induced lupus:

- Acecainide
- Allopurinol
- Aminogluthimide
- Amoproxam
- Anthiomaline
- Anti-tumor necrosis factor-alpha
- Benoxaprofen
- Captopril
- Chlorprothixene
- Cimetidine
- Cinnarizine
- Clonidine
- Danazol
- Diclofenac
- Diphenylhydantoin
- D-penicillamine
- Enalapril
- Estrogens
- Ethosuximide

- Ethylphenacemide
- Gold salts
- Griseofulvin
- Guanoxan
- Ibuprofen
- Interferon-alpha and gamma
- Interleukin-2
- Leuprolide acetate
- Levoadopa (L-Dopa)
- Lithium carbonate
- Lovastatin
- Mephenytoin
- Methimazole
- Metrizamide
- Minoxidil
- Nalicidic acid
- Nitrofurantoin
- Oxyprenolol
- Penicillin
- Phenazine
- Prazosin
- Promethazine
- Quinine
- Reserpine
- Simvastatin
- Spironolactone
- Streptomycin
- Sulfadimethoxine
- Sulfasalazine
- Sulindac
- Tetracyclines

- Tetrazine
- Thionamide
- Thioridazine
- Timolol eye drops
- Tolazamide
- Tolmetin
- Trimethadione.

Environmental chemicals, heavy metals, dietary factors: Agents associated with lupus-like syndrome also include environmental chemicals, heavy metals, certain foods, hydrazine (present in tobacco, penicillin, mushrooms, and several agricultural and industrial compounds).

Tartrazine and paraphenylenediamine (present in some dyes, such as the azo food and hair dyes) are chemical agents that may induce the syndrome. Among the heavy metals, mercury, gold, cadmium, lithium, chromium, and zinc have been implicated in producing autoimmune diseases and lupus-like syndrome. Metals that have been associated with other autoimmune diseases are silica, silicon, and vinyl chloride. Industrial solvents are also especially suspected. Long-term exposures to chemicals in computer manufacturing, industrial emissions, and hazardous waste have been reported in drug-induced lupus studies.

The following food and dietary factors have been cited as causing lupus-like syndrome or activation of systemic lupus:

- Some tests suggest that toxic substances in water, such as trichloroethylene found in some well water, may trigger the syndrome.
- L-canavanine is an amino acid present in sprouts and alfalfa seeds that may cause drug-induced lupus or

activation of the disease in patients with systemic lupus. It can also cause hemolytic anemia. Discontinuation of its use reverses the symptoms.

• Anilines, chemicals related to benzene, and L-tryptophan have been implicated as possible factors inducing adverse autoimmune effects. In one report, when anilines were used to denature rapeseed (canola) oil, individuals using the oil developed acute pneumonitis, scleroderma-like skin disease (loss of elasticity of the skin), neuromyopathy, (disorder of the nerves and associated muscle tissue), and Sjögren's syndrome (an autoimmune disease), all of which were attributed to toxic oil syndrome.

In another report, L-tryptophan, which is an essential amino acid, caused similar problems to those of aniline, but the disease mechanism is not clear. Individuals taking L-tryptophan as a dietary supplement developed elevated type of white blood cells (eosinophils) and, in some cases, were also antinuclear antibody positive.

Viruses: Several viral infections may be associated with lupus, but study results have not confirmed this. Some of the viruses suspected to have a relationship with lupus are the following:

• Human herpes virus (HPV)
• Parvovirus
• Measles
• Mumps
• Myxoviruses (a variant of the influenza virus)
• Retroviruses
• Oncornaviruses.

Because of the association of these and other viruses with lupus, live vaccines with attenuated organisms are not advisable. Lupus patients need to consult their physicians before receiving any type of immunization. However, lupus patients who have been exposed to viral infections (such as chicken pox or measles) but who have not acquired immunity either by a vaccine or the disease itself need to notify their physicians immediately to undergo preventive or protective therapy. Most of these therapies need to be administered within the first 72 hours after exposure to the offending organism. Otherwise, patients should be observed for signs of disease development and receive specific therapy as needed.

Researchers across the world continue to study the role that environmental triggers may play in the development of lupus.

CHAPTER NINE

﹙❧﹚

CURRENT RESEARCH

M EDICAL RESEARCHERS are continually working to learn more about lupus. Research in the last decade has greatly improved our understanding. Several environmental and genetic factors are thought to predispose an individual to the development of lupus. Since the environmental factors have already been discussed, let's discuss the genetic factors. Convincing evidence suggests that lupus is a genetic disorder. Studies show 7–12 percent of lupus patients have a first- and second-degree relative with lupus. About 60 percent of identical twins and 2–5 percent of non-identical twins and other siblings will share the disease. Interestingly, other autoimmune diseases and serologic (blood test) abnormalities are also present at a high frequency in the families of lupus patients, which also suggests an underlying genetic predisposition to autoimmune diseases.

To understand the meaning of the genetic predisposition, it is important to understand the terms. Genetics is the study of the genes, which are found only in living cells. These are often called the "blueprints" of the cells. Each gene contains the "recipe" for the specific function and development of the cells. Everyone has his or her own unique set of genes, or genetic code (collection of genes within a cell). This means that the genetic code of your parents or siblings is different from yours. This is why every person in the same family is different, with different physical characteristics such as hair color, eyes, and body shape.

The human body is made up of trillions of living cells of various types. Each cell has a specialized function in the body. For example, there are brain cells, heart cells, skin cells, bone cells, and many other types of cells. Because of the multiple functions the cell has to perform, each cell has different components inside it, just like a car. For your car to work, it has to have an engine, oil, gas, wheels, and so on. Thus, all the different parts of the cell are contained within what is called the cell membrane. The nucleus, an essential component of the cell, is the cell's "control center." The nucleus is like the car engine; without a good engine, the car won't work. The genes are located inside the nucleus and contain of all of the instructions required to make the chemicals and proteins essential for life.

Genes are shorter segments of long molecules called DNA (deoxyribonucleic acid) that store the cell's specific and unique hereditary characteristics. Genes are connected with each other in patterns or sequences called linkage. The particular order of this linkage predisposes each of us to inherit certain characteristics. Genes are coiled in spooled-up strands of DNA called chromosomes within the cell's nucleus. Chromosomes carry genetic information that shapes us. Each of the trillions of cells in the human body has a complete set of chromosomes, called a genome. The human genome contains more than 30,000 genes. A human cell has a total of 46 chromosomes (23 almost identical pairs, one set inherited from each parent).

DNA is made up of four different chemical bases, or building blocks, known as amino acids. Comprised of protein, these chemical bases are adenine, cytosine, guanine, and thymine. DNA contains billions of these amino acids in different orders to create libraries of genetic information in the nuclei of our cells. A genome can be compared to a huge library full of information. These chemical libraries are formed from subunits of information, where the bases (amino acids) are like letters of the alphabet, genes are entire sections of the library, and chromosomes are complete floors of a 23-story library.

In summary, thousands of genes join together in a chain-like formation to make a DNA molecule, and two DNA strands wound together form a chromosome (hence the term "double-stranded DNA molecule"). Every one of us has 46 chromosomes (2 sets of 23), each of which is composed of thousands of genes (see Figure 9) and usually collected in the nucleus of each of the body's cells.

Genes have different characteristics, and some are "stronger" than others. Dominant genes are those that are stronger and result in the dominant inheritance characteristics. Genes that are "weaker" represent the recessive inheritance, which are characteristics that appear less often. However, even though genes provide the instructions for the cell, the intended functions do not always occur.

This malfunction may be the result of other factors influencing the cells, such as the environment, injuries, poor nutrition, and other behavioral factors. Another factor that can cause cellular changes is called a *mutation*, which is a rare and random "mistake" in the DNA. Genetic diseases may be caused by mutations. A different, more common variation of a gene is called a polymorphism.

Figure 9. Human Chromosome

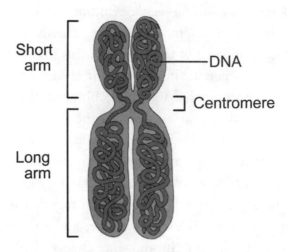

Genes are studied to learn about their effects in an individual or in a family. The outcome or visible result that characterizes any specific gene is called a phenotype, whereas the genotype is the genetic makeup of an individual.

For example, say a specific gene can *encode* (provide instructions for) for black hair; then that is your genotype for hair color. The black hair itself is the phenotype, the end product that you can see.

In studying the particular genetic makeup of a family, researchers look at the phenotypes among family members to reveal information about the genotypes, or the genetic makeup of that particular family. Because humans have numerous traits, the study of their genotypes can be quite complicated. One of the first things that the investigator or researcher does as part of the investigation of the family is to interview individual family members to gather specific information about family history and conditions. This information helps explain how the specific trait or traits are passed along from generation to generation.

This is easily visualized by drawing a family tree or a pedigree diagram (see Figure 10). This type of study is used to study the origin of various diseases, including lupus. Although there have been many advances in genetic research, much more is needed to help us understand diseases, especially the complex autoimmune diseases. Several genetic linkages have been discovered in the search for the specific gene or genes that may cause lupus or its complications. More than twenty of these linkages have been found so far. Based on preliminary studies, there seems to be more than one gene that causes lupus. Some of the genes that predispose one to lupus may vary by race, but other genes may be common to different races. The genes may be influential in determining the type and severity of lupus. There also may be genes specific to kidney disease, hemolytic anemia, arthritis, and

Figure 10. Pedigree Diagram

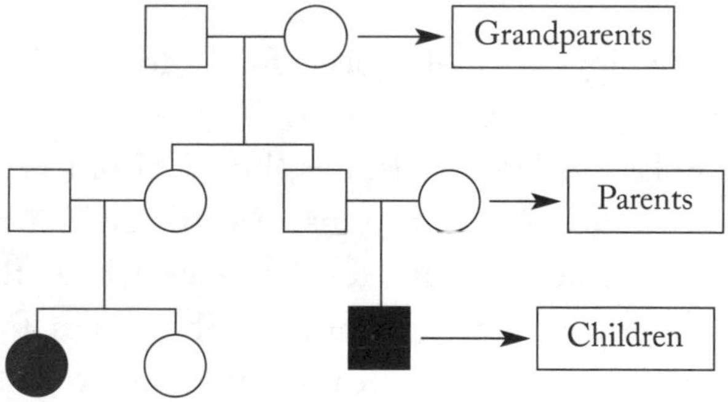

This is an example of a family tree or pedigree diagram. The circles represent the females, and the squares represent the males. Married men and women are connected by horizontal lines. The diagram starts with the oldest generation at the top, followed below by each succeeding generation. The most recent generation is at the bottom of the figure. Once all the figures or family members are added to the diagram, traits of interest are recorded. For example, in this figure we have two affected patients with lupus. More than one trait can be recorded on the same pedigree diagram.

other systemic manifestations of lupus. The identification of the lupus genes may one day permit us to correct genetic defects through therapy and improve disease prognosis.

Lupus shows itself differently among the various ethnic groups, and this fact may account for the differences in survival rates. Studies suggest that African Americans have a higher incidence of kidney disease, low white blood cells (leukopenia and lymphopenia), hair loss, muscle inflammation, and the presence of anti-Smith and anti-nRNP autoantibodies (see Chapter 3). Another study showed that Hispanics, followed by European Americans, are more inclined to have malar rash and photosensitivity.

Other research found that African Americans with lupus present less frequently with Sjögren's syndrome, antiphospholipid antibodies, anti-cardiolipin, and lupus anticoagulant than do European Americans. African-American patients may also have a more active disease course at an earlier age of onset than do European Americans.

Genetic findings have also been found for specific clinical manifestations in lupus. Certain areas of different chromosomes have been linked to kidney diseases, blood disorders, arthritis, vitiligo, and other complications. Most locations in the chromosome have been specific for each race, while others have been seen in general. For example, possible genes for kidney disease have been found in an area of chromosome 10 for white lupus patients but in another area of chromosome 2 for black patients. Such discoveries are helping us discover new gene therapies to prevent or cure specific complications that cause so many problems in lupus patients.

Other studies have investigated the relationship between lupus and birth order. It has been found that there is a 50 percent risk of having lupus among firstborns, compared to a lower risk in second borns, and a much lower risk among subsequent births.

CLINICAL TRIALS

In clinical trials (studies conducted with patients' participation), research scientists study new therapies that could control or cure diseases. Lupus patients are encouraged to participate in clinical trials and other ongoing research. Participating in trials may help the patient personally, as well as help scientists discover how lupus starts, how it develops, and new ways to detect and treat it. New information may lead to new methods for preventing the occurrence of lupus. Information on how and where you may participate in lupus research can be obtained from Chapter 10, as well as from your physician, the Internet, and the media.

There are a few things you should know if you are considering participating in a clinical study. Above all, your participation in any medical study is voluntary. Once you decide to participate, the investigator or the study coordinator will explain to you in detail what the study is about, what will be required of you, and any complications that may arise from the study. The coordinator will also explain your rights as a study participant. In some genetic studies, your family will be asked to participate, so they too may need to be educated about the study. Once you and perhaps your family members agree to participate, you will be asked to sign a consent form attesting to the fact that you understand your obligations as a participant and the possible benefits and risks The consent agreement is essential for your participation in any study. This document will authorize the investigator to use your samples and any information gathered in the research being conducted. If you do not sign the consent agreement, the investigator is prohibited by law to use your samples or information.

Most consent agreements will include the following sections: the purpose of the study, the procedures involved, confidentiality of your personal information, the cost (if any) of participating, contact information of the investigator and the Institution Review Board (IRB), and where the study takes place.

The procedure section of the consent agreement will include information related to what types of samples are required for participation. If blood samples are to be taken, the amount of blood required as well as the times that the procedure needs to be repeated should be specified. A repeated procedure usually indicates that the investigators and your doctor believe there is additional information that should be reported to you or the public. In addition, the form should specify where the samples are going to be kept and how are they going to be used. Your samples may be tested immediately, or they may be frozen and used for later tests.

Your samples will be stored not by your name but with a confidential code. Samples may be kept until no cells, serum, plasma, or DNA remain, or until the investigators decide to destroy them. Sometimes, the samples may be released to other doctors and medical scientists who are not associated with the institution conducting the study. Their research may reveal different or additional information about lupus that may aid the original investigator. You will not be asked to sign another consent form for future uses of your samples provided that your privacy can be assured in these other studies. If you or the new investigators suspect that there are any risks to your privacy, you should be asked to sign another consent agreement for new uses of your samples. The investigators in charge of the new study will determine exactly how and in what center your samples will be used. Regardless, any study must have been approved by the Institutional Review Board; this group exists primarily to ensure that patients' rights are respected in all research activities.

As a participant, your private personal information (such as name, address, telephone number) will be kept separately from the results of research tests performed on your samples. All of the research information should be kept in a password-protected computer file that only the investigators and their staff can access. You may be asked to complete other documents, such as a questionnaire concerning your medical history and other related information required for the study. Some studies may require access to your medical records. However, you will need to authorize the use of those records by signing a release form, and if you do so, your information will be kept strictly confidential.

The risks of any research study will depend on the type of investigation being conducted. For example, if participating in the study requires providing a blood sample, then the risk might be discomfort, bleeding, or bruising at the site of injection. Donating blood might also result in dizziness or fainting. On the rare occasions that a nonsterile needle is used, an infection may develop at the site where the blood was collected. Other possible risks include the research not resulting in new, useful information or perhaps an unauthorized person may review your confidential information. Under certain circumstances, research records, like hospital records, can be requested by court order. In such rare cases, your complete privacy and the privacy of other family members participating in the research cannot be guaranteed. However, prior to the start of the study, the investigator can request a Certificate of Confidentiality from the U.S. Department of Health and Human Services for "Genetic Studies"; this document will protect the privacy of research subjects by withholding their identities from all persons not connected with the research.

If you prefer to discontinue your participation in the research, you may request that any samples you donated be destroyed. At that point, you should not be asked for further information or samples and your identity should be removed from all research records. However, neither the resulting data from the study nor any cell lines previously obtained will be destroyed.

You have the right to agree or refuse to participate in any type of research. If you decide to participate you should be free to withdraw at any time during the study. Refusal to participate will not result in penalty or loss of your entitled benefits nor will it affect your legal rights or the quality of healthcare that you will receive at the center where the study is conducted. You will be updated on any new information that may become available during the study that may affect your willingness to continue participating.

Remember that you have the right to privacy. All of your private information obtained from the research should remain confidential within the limits of the law. You should be assured that neither you nor your family members will be identifiable by name in any reports or publications that may result from the study.

WES'S STORY

It's like it was yesterday, yet it's been over twelve years since I was diagnosed with lupus. It happened so quickly. I was a solider at the time, preparing my unit to go to war, and, almost at the next moment,

I'm on my deathbed! In only three months I went from being a healthy thirty-one-year-old man to someone who couldn't even feed himself.

How did it change my life? The worst was the loss of physical abilities. Not being able to put on clothes, not enough strength to tie my shoes, and worst of all, not being able to go to the bathroom without help. As the medications started to work, things did become better but I still had to put up with constant pain and the fear that, yes, I could die. The fear that the medications will not work during a flare-up is always there.

I have two kids who couldn't recognize me when I was in the hospital; they were actually afraid at first! I often think of the things I could do with my kids before, like playing or baseball—which I can no longer do.

Even my career changed. My friends in the military are all retiring with a rank of Lt. Colonel or higher, but my opportunity was taken away from me by lupus. The military had to run several thousands of dollars of tests just to figure out what was wrong with me in the beginning—which only added to the frustration. The drugs I had to take changed my life as well as my personality. I had no confidence that I could or would ever find anybody who would want to be with me. I was divorced and alone and couldn't date.

What did I do to adapt to my new life? When I was in the hospital I would joke around; I soon found the laughter helped. A lot of other things contributed to my getting better—a belief in God, trust in the doctors, consistently taking the medications that stop the disease process, and, most of all, my own desire to stay around awhile.

I even found positive things about my disease. I have been given the ability to help others understand the disease. I stopped being a workaholic. I learned to adapt to the physical changes by finding other ways to get around. I now can relate better to people. I've even become more patient with my kids and understand their needs better. My confidence with the opposite sex is improving and the best yet: I regularly give samples of blood for research. Who knows? My blood might actually be critical in finding a cure!

>—•

CHAPTER TEN

>❦

PATIENTS' RESOURCES

I N THIS CHAPTER, you will find numerous resources available for obtaining information and assistance. These include how to seek medical assistance, Internet sites of different organizations related to lupus, and a group of selected publications that will broaden your knowledge about the disease.

HOW TO SEEK MEDICAL ASSISTANCE

It is very important that everyone has a primary care physician, and this is especially true of lupus patients. A primary care physician coordinates your healthcare with other physicians as needed, including any tests that need to be performed or specialists that need to be consulted. Patients can find a primary care physician through their health insurance company's directory of physicians or perhaps through referrals from other patients. Those patients who do not have insurance and cannot afford to go to a private doctor may seek help from free clinics in their communities. These clinics usually are run through a government agency or through a program set up by charitable organizations. You can usually find information about these clinics from your community leaders, medical society, or government agencies.

I cannot overemphasize the importance of coordinating medical services when someone has a disease such as lupus that can affect many organ systems. Perhaps the most important thing in getting excellent medical care is to have a caring and involved primary care provider (PCP) who communicates with the specialists involved in your care. It will be that primary care provider who will see you first when problems arise, and the primary care provider will work closely with you to prevent problems in the first place. Most people with lupus will need the expertise of subspecialists to help diagnose and manage their disease. Rheumatologists, nephrologists (kidney specialists), cardiologists, neurologists, gastroenterologists, orthopedists, and transplant surgeons are commonly consulted for patients with lupus. Though most people will not need all these specialists, one or more may be involved in your care at some time. It is important that each physician communicate with each other, and also with your primary care provider, who links all the services together and functions as the patient's advocate in the complex healthcare networks.

When more than one specialist is involved, it becomes even more important to be sure that they communicate with each other. I have seen situations where a patient is taking a drug prescribed by the primary care provider, and another brand of the same drug prescribed by the kidney doctor, for example. The best way to avoid this is to bring all your medicine bottles to all your doctor visits and to ask each doctor to send notes to all the other physicians involved in your care. Be sure they have the correct names and addresses of each one. Coordination of care is increasingly important as the number of healthcare providers increases. Don't leave anything to chance. Get yourself a good primary care provider, be sure all specialists send notes to each other, and always review every medication you are taking at each doctor visit. Don't leave anything to chance!

M. O'Neil, M.D.
Pediatric Rheumatologist

}~

Once you have selected a primary care physician, you will need to tell him or her about any health problems that you may have. Primary care for children is often provided by pediatricians or, in some cases, by the family doctor. Primary care for adults is usually provided by the family doctor, a general physician, or an internist.

Patients covered by an insurance plan can contact their insurance company, which will provide a directory of physicians who accept their particular insurance plan. In some instances, the insurance company will ask you to call the physician directly to investigate whether he or she accepts your insurance coverage, and if not, accepts private patients. Private patients are usually those who do not have insurance and, because of their income level, do not qualify for the special clinics or services offered through the government, including Medicaid or Medicare insurance.

If the patient needs to be seen by a specialist (a doctor who is dedicated to the care of specific area of the body or special conditions, like the rheumatologist), the primary care physician will provide a referral. For example, lupus patients are often referred to a rheumatologist who specializes in the care of patients with lupus, arthritis, dermatomyositis (systemic inflammatory muscle disease), and other rheumatologic conditions. The rheumatologist will then coordinate the care of the lupus patient with the primary care physician. Other specialists may need to be involved in your care as well. This all will depend on the symptoms and needs that you may have.

MANAGING YOUR MEDICAL CARE

Healthcare can be very costly, especially for chronic diseases like lupus, but there are many programs that can help you obtain what you need to continue your care. Some of these programs are offered by pharmaceutical companies that help qualified patients obtain medications at discounted rates. Not all pharmaceutical companies offer these programs however, and not all the medicines are covered by the programs that are offered. Later in this chapter, you will find a list of some of these pharmaceutical companies and the medical programs that they offer.

Some patients may encounter problems with their employer because of a large number of absences from work due to illness. You should talk to your supervisor to see if it is possible to make special arrangements. If this is not possible because of the type of work or the regulations of the company, then you might try to find another work situation that can better accommodate your personal or health-related needs.

Other patients may become incapacitated by secondary complications of lupus for which they may be able to apply for disability compensation. A listing of contact information is available later in this chapter under the heading "U.S. Government Web Sites." If you believe you are a candidate to receive disability payments, you should contact the nearest office and request all pertinent information. Disability, as defined by the Social Security Administration, is the inability to engage in any substantial, gainful activity because of physical or mental impairment that has lasted or can be expected to last for a continuous period of more than twelve months or that can be expected to result in death. In other words, disability is your inability to work. The Social Security Administration recognizes lupus as a potentially disabling illness and it is included in their listing of impairments.

The process of filing for disability insurance and receiving a response from the Social Security Disability Insurance can take a long time. For some, the process can take a year or more, resulting in a very stressful situation. Consequently, it may be beneficial to have family members or friends help you with the paperwork and keep track of your appointments. Some patients may even need the help of an attorney in negotiating the many documents required. If you do request the assistance of an attorney, confirm that this person is knowledgeable about all the rules, regulations, and procedures of the Social Security Administration. Be advised that in some cases, disability claims are rejected on the first application and you may need to reapply. It will be wise to have your medical records and statements from your physician, supervisor, or coworkers available to facilitate the process. To confirm your disability, the Social Security agency may require a physical exam by one of their doctors. Do not give up; be persistent if you believe you qualify for the services. It is wise to stay current with the most recent information, because the rules can change at any time.

Learning to control lupus is very challenging for both the patient and family. A plan of treatment that includes therapy, medication, and doctors' visits may place a strain on the family financially, especially if the patient has no medical insurance.

Working with "rheumatology children" can be challenging in numerous ways. I saw a fifteen-year-old girl with lupus who had been hospitalized for two weeks and part of that time she was in the intensive care unit. While in our office, her mother said she'd never heard of lupus until she was told her daughter might have it, and just the word "lupus" scared her. Then her daughter was hospitalized with hemolytic anemia and part of that time she was in the intensive care unit, she was even more scared.

Now that she's home they have another fear, that is, how they will buy her medications and pay for the rheumatologist to continue to care for her or anything else she needs to treat her lupus. She'd discussed this with others and had been informed that their family income exceeded that allowed for her daughter to qualify for state medical insurance. By trial and error she and I checked out a number of ideas and through sheer determination we found a solution to assist with all bills related to her lupus. This took less than a month to accomplish. Two years later she got medical insurance.

My role as their nurse includes ensuring that patients will have access to wherever resources they need to treat their lupus. I let them know that there are resources we can use should they encounter obstacles such as getting their insurance to pay for needed medications, or if they don't have insurance. Community resources and pharmaceutical companies have helped a number of our patients.

Linda Menifee, R.N.
Rheumatology Nurse

❧

PATIENTS' RIGHTS

As previously explained, the privacy of patients' health information is protected by federal law. Research on patients is primarily regulated by the Department of Health and Human Services (HHS), which requires a research study to have the approval of the Institutional Review Board to conduct federally funded biomedical research. The Federal Drug Administration (FDA), the Public Health Service, and various state laws also regulate this research. However, privately funded research is not subject to Institutional Review Board requirements. Yet effective April 2003, federal law requires the creation and use of a board to administer the privacy requirements under what is called the HIPAA rules.

HIPAA stands for Health Insurance Portability and Accountability Act. This is a series of rules created in 1996 by the Department of Health and Human Services to protect patients' privacy rights. These rules apply to your physicians and other healthcare providers involved in your care. HIPAA bars disclosure of information for reasons unrelated to healthcare unless the patient gives permission. Hospitals will no longer release information about a patient's condition or even confirm that the person is a patient unless the patient agrees to be listed in the hospital's directory. This new regulation provides patients with access to their medical records and gives them more control over how their personal health information is used and disclosed. The HIPAA Act represents a much more uniform privacy protection standard for patients across the country.

These new privacy regulations apply at a national level but they do not affect state laws that provide additional privacy protections for patients. The privacy protections for patients limit the ways that health plans, pharmacies, hospitals, and other covered entities can use patients' personal medical information. Medical records and other individually identifiable health information are now legally protected, whether the information is on paper, in computers, or communicated orally. Patients should be able to see and obtain copies of their medical records and request corrections if they identify errors. Covered health plans, doctors, and other healthcare providers must provide a notice to their patients on how they may use personal medical information and their rights under the new privacy regulation. Doctors, hospitals, and other direct-care providers will generally provide the notice on the patient's first visit. Patients will be asked to sign that they have received this notice.

The Privacy Rule sets limits on how health plans and covered providers may use individually identifiable health information. To promote the best quality of care for patients, the rule does not restrict the ability of doctors, nurses, and other providers to share information needed to treat their patients. In addition, patients would have to sign a specific authorization to allow release of their medical information to a life insurance company, a bank, a marketing firm, or other outside businesses for purposes not related to their health care. Patients can request that all "covered entities" (such as doctors, health plans, and pharmacists) take reasonable steps to ensure that their communications with the patient are confidential. The rules also place limits on the use of the patient's information for marketing purposes. Anyone disclosing a patient's information for marketing purposes must first obtain an individual's specific authorization to do so. Further, the covered entities must train their employees in their privacy procedures and must designate an individual to be responsible for ensuring that the procedures are followed.

Congress imposes civil and criminal penalties for covered entities that misuse personal health information. For civil violations of the standards, fines can be up to $100 per violation, or up to $25,000 per year. Criminal penalties apply to those who knowingly obtain protected health information in violation of the law, with fines up to $50,000 and prison sentences up to one year for certain offenses. If the criminal offense is committed under "false pretenses," the penalty can be a fine up to $100,000 and up to five years in prison. If the offense is committed with the intent to sell, transfer, or use protected health information for commercial advantage, personal gain, or malicious harm, the penalty can be a fine up to $250,000 and up to ten years in prison.

Patients who believe that their rights have been violated can file a Health Information Privacy Complaint with the Office for Civil Rights (OCR). If a person, agency, or organization covered under the HIPAA Privacy Rule committed any violation of the Privacy Rule, a complaint may be filed with the Office for Civil Rights. The Office for Civil Rights receives and investigates complaints against covered entities related to the Privacy Rule. Complaints to the Office for Civil Rights must be filed in writing, either on paper or electronically, including the name of the entity that is the subject of the complaint and a description of the acts or omissions believed to be in violation of the Privacy Rule (that occurred on or after April 14, 2003, when the law went into effect). The complaint should be filed within 180 days of when the alleged violation or omission came into question. You can contact the Office for Civil Rights regarding questions about the complaint form or procedures at their toll-free number: 800–368–1019, or go to their Web site at *www.hhs.gov/ocr/privacyhowtofile.htm*.

INTERNET INFORMATION ON LUPUS AND RELATED DISORDERS

There is a great deal of information on the Internet about lupus, but not all the information available will apply to you and much may prove to be unreliable. Following is a list of recommended Web sites.

National Organizations

Lupus Foundation of America
2000 L Street, NW, Suite 710
Washington, DC 20036
Ph: 202–349–1155
www.lupus.org

Lupus Foundation of America (LFA) is a nonprofit voluntary organization dedicated to finding the cause and cure for lupus. The LFA has fifty chapters with hundreds of support groups across the nation. The LFA supports individuals and families affected by the disease and seeks to increase awareness of lupus among health professionals and the public. Research, education, and patient services are at the heart of LFA's programs. The Web site also includes information about support groups across the nation.

Lupus Alliance of America
3871 Harlem Road
Buffalo, NY 14215
Ph: 1–866–415–8787
www.lupusalliance.org

The Lupus Alliance of America is composed of affiliated member groups across the country. The Alliance provides support and educational material to their affiliates and the public in an effort to enhance services to the lupus community.

Arthritis Foundation
National Office
1330 West Peachtree Street
Atlanta, GA 30309
www.arthritis.org

The Arthritis Foundation is composed of health professionals and individual members. The Foundation provides information, activities, and the latest research news on arthritis and related diseases. The Arthritis Foundation has multiple chapters across the nation.

Ohio Chapters of the Lupus Foundation of America
Chapter in Central Ohio
6161 Busch Blvd., Suite 76
Columbus, OH 43229
Ph: 614–846–9249 or 614–221 0811 (hotline)
www.lupusohio.org

This Web site provides information about lupus, online support groups, and other related topics for lupus patients.

The Texas Gulf Coast Chapter of the Lupus Foundation of
    America
3730 Kirby Drive, Suite 720
Houston, TX 77098–3927
Ph: 713–529–0126 or 800–458–7870 (toll-free)
www.lupustexas.org

This Web site offers information about lupus, its diagnosis and treatment, and support groups for individuals and families affected by the disease.

Antiphospholipid Syndrome
www.neuroland.com/cvd/aps.htm

This Web site provides a variety of information about lupus and its complications such as the involvement of the central nervous system.

Johns Hopkins Vasculitis Center
c/o Dr. John Stone
Bayview Medical Center
5501 Hopkins Bayview Circle
JHAAC, Room 1B.1A
Baltimore, MD 21224
Ph: 410–550–6816
http://vasculitis.med.jhu.edu

This Web site provides information about vasculitis, the Vaculitis Center's facilities and personnel, and where to find additional resources. In addition, there is information about research studies on vasculitis in which patients can participate.

Community, Information, Resources on Diseases Disorders and
    Chronic Illnesses
www.healingwell.com

This Web site provides information for patients, caregivers, and families coping with diseases, disorders, and chronic illness. You will find medical news, feature articles, doctor-produced videos, message boards, chat rooms, e-mail addresses, health e-greeting cards, newsletters, books and reviews, and a resource directory.

Lupus Links
www.sblupus.org/lupuslinks.html

This Web page offers a large number of other Web site addresses about lupus and its related disorders, and patients' stories about living with lupus.

Black Women's Health

www.blackwomenshealth.com/lupus.htm

This Web site is dedicated to promoting the physical, mental, and spiritual wellness of African-American women. You will find information about lupus and other conditions, as well as a medical directory to help you find a physician near you, events, and other support material.

Results About Lupus

http://results.about.com/lupus/

This Web site offers links to information related to lupus, including research, support groups, and other associations with the shared goal of helping patients with autoimmune disorders.

Skin Disease in Lupus - Lupus Profundis

www.hamline.edu/lupus/articles/skin_disease_in_lupus.html

This Web page will give you more information of the skin manifestations of lupus.

Lupus Beacon
L. E. Support Club
8039 Nova Court
North Charleston, SC 29420–8934
E-mail: hbmesic@knology.net
www.galaxymall.com/commerce/lupus/index.html

This Web site provides a newsletter with the latest information for lupus patients, other resources, testimonials, and support groups.

Lupus Listserv Group
www.acor.org/lupus

This is a listserv group that addresses the need for sharing information and support for systemic lupus erythematosus, discoid lupus, and related diseases. A listserv group is an Internet communication tool that offers its members the opportunity to post suggestions or questions to a large number of people at the same time. When you submit a question or information to share to the listserv, your submission is distributed to all of the members on that list.

Center Watch
22 Thomson Place, 36T1
Boston, MA 02210–1212
Ph: 617–856–5900
www.centerwatch.com

This Boston–based publishing and information services company provides information services used by patients; pharmaceutical, biotechnology, and medical device companies; and research centers involved in clinical research around the world.

American Medical Association
515 N. State Street
Chicago, IL 60610
Ph: 800–621–8335 (toll-free)
www.ama-assn.org

The American Medical Association (AMA) is one of the largest medical associations in the world. The AMA is an actively lobbies Congress for the benefit of the public health. The AMA Web site provides health information, doctor-finder information, and books for patients.

Rheuma21st

www.rheuma21st.com

*This Web site provides news of important developments in
rheumatology and immunology prior to their publication in print
journals. The Web site editors are a group of academic and practicing
rheumatologists and immunologists from all over the world who are
among the leading teaching experts in their fields. They select
information from closed or little-known meetings that discuss the
latest developments in their respective areas.*

American Autoimmune Related Diseases Association National
    Office
22100 Gratiot Avenue
E. Detroit, MI 48021
Ph: 810–776–3900
www.aarda.org

*This is a nonprofit health agency dedicated to the eradication of
autoimmune diseases through fostering and facilitating collaboration
in the areas of education, public awareness, research, and patient
services. The Web site provides information about a variety of
autoimmune diseases.*

Family Caregiver Alliance
690 Market Street, Suite 600
San Francisco, CA 94104
Ph: 415–434–3388 or 800–445–8106 (toll-free)
www.caregiver.org

*This Web site offers information on materials widely utilized by
caregivers and resources about the innovative services for families*

*and professional care providers. Families can call the toll-free number
to request advice.*

Systemic Lupus Erythematosus in Pediatrics
E-mail: jeg@sbceo.org
www.kidlupus.org

*This Web site offers information related to lupus in children,
recommendations, and resources.*

Lupus Erythematosus
National Office
2000 L Street, N.W., Suite 710
Washington, DC 20036
Ph: 202–349–1155
Ph: 800–558–0121 (Information request line)
Ph: 800–558–0231 (Para información en Español) (Spanish)
www.familyvillage.wisc.edu/lib_lups.htm

*This Web site is a family lupus chat room originated by the Lupus
Foundation of America.*

Specialty Organizations and Associations
American College of Rheumatology
1800 Century Place, Suite 250
Atlanta, GA 30345–4300
Ph: 404 633 3777
www.rheumatology.org

*This is a professional organization of rheumatologists and associated
health professionals who share a dedication to healing, preventing
disability, and curing the more than 100 types of arthritis and
related rheumatologic conditions. It offers a directory of*

rheumatologists and rheumatology health professionals. It also provides information about the latest legislation that affects patient care, federal funding of rheumatology research, and a variety of services for its members and the public. In addition, the site includes links to other subject areas related to rheumatic diseases.

The American Academy of Dermatology
P.O. Box 4014
Schaumburg, IL 60168–4014
Ph: 847–330–0230
www.aad.org

This organization is dedicated on achieving the highest quality of dermatologic care for everyone and offers a variety of information and education for patients and health professionals.

The American Academy of Neurology
1080 Montreal Avenue
Saint Paul, MN 55116
Ph: (800) 879–1960 or (651) 695–2717
www.aan.com/professionals

The American Academy of Neurology is an international association of neurologists and neuroscience professionals dedicated to providing the best care to patients with neurological disorders. It offers patient orientation and information on the latest discoveries in neurology.

American Academy of Ophthalmology
P.O. Box 7424
San Francisco, CA 94120–7424
Ph: 415.561.8500
www.aao.org

The American Academy of Ophthalmology is the largest national membership association of eye specialists. The Web site includes a medical library, medical news, and learning center.

American Society of Nephrology
1725 I Street, NW, Suite 510
Washington, DC   20006
Ph: 202–659–0599
www.asn-online.org

The American Society of Nephrology is a nonprofit corporation that enhances and assists the study and practice of nephrology, provides a forum for the promulgation of research, and meets the professional and continuing education needs of its members. The Web site provides links to the latest information related to kidney diseases.

National Sleep Association
1522 K Street, NW, Suite 500
Washington, DC 20005
Ph: 202–347–3471
www.sleepfoundation.org

This organization provides information to improve the quality of life for people who suffer from sleep problems and disorders. The Web site provides information that will help you understand better the importance of sleep, practice good sleep habits, and recognize the signs of sleep problems so that they can be properly diagnosed and treated. The organization offers public education and participates in awareness initiatives, government relations, advocacy efforts, and support for further research.

American Dietetic Association
120 South Riverside Plaza, Suite 2000
Chicago, IL 60606–6995
Ph: 800–877–1600
www.eatright.org

This is one of the nation's largest organizations of food and nutrition professionals. It addresses issues such as children's health, food technology and safety, public health, consumer education, healthcare reform, nutrition for the elderly, and healthcare provider education.

American Psychological Association
750 First Street NE
Washington, DC 20002–4242
Ph: 800–964–2000
http://apahelpcenter.org

This Web site offers a directory for locating psychologists in your area. In addition, there is a variety of information on different aspects of psychological problems and support. The site also provides information about the wide range of legislative and regulatory issues of interest to the organization.

American Pain Foundation
Ph: 888–615–PAIN (7246)
www.painfoundation.org

This is an independent nonprofit organization serving people with pain by offering information, advocacy, and support. Its mission is to improve the quality of life of people with pain by raising public awareness, providing practical information, promoting research, and increasing access to effective pain management.

American Lung Association
Ph: 800–LUNG-USA (800–586–4872)
www.lungusa.org

The mission of the American Lung Association is to fight lung disease in all its forms, with special emphasis on asthma, tobacco control, and environmental health.

Myositis Association of America
1233 20th Street NW, Suite 402
Washington, DC 20036
Ph: 202–887–0088
www.myositis.org

This organization provides a range of programs and services to those concerned about myositis. It provides and communicates timely information, research updates, and funding opportunities to health professionals and offers referral to support groups for their patients. It supports patients and families with informative newsletters, conferences, updates, and support groups. It also offers children's programs to address the specific needs of families dealing with myositis.

National Kidney Foundation
30 East 33rd Street, Suite 1100
New York, NY 10016
Ph: 800–622–9010 or 212–889–2210
www.kidney.org

This is a voluntary health organization that seeks to prevent kidney and urinary tract diseases, improve the health and well-being of individuals and families affected by these diseases, and increase the availability of all organs for transplantation.

Nova Online

www.pbs.org/wgbh/nova/heart

This Web site provides information about the heart and the many conditions that may affect it. It also offers several links to other Web sites that are resources on heart conditions.

National Stroke Association
9707 E. Easter Lane
Englewood, CO 80112
Ph: 1–800–STROKES
Ph: 303–649–9299

www.stroke.org

This organization provides expertise and leadership for those at risk, suffering, or recovering from strokes. It seeks to educate the public about the steps that can be taken to reduce the incidence and impact of strokes.

Pulmonary Hypertension Association
850 Sligo Avenue, Suite 800
Silver Spring, MD 20910
Ph: 301–565–3004 or 800–748–7274

www.phassociation.org

This Web site provides information on support groups, promotes public awareness and education programs, and advocates for the pulmonary hypertension community.

Sjögren's Syndrome Foundation
8120 Woodmont Avenue, Suite 530
Bethesda, MD 20814
Ph: 800–475–6473 (voice mail only)

www.sjogrens.org

The Sjögren's Syndrome Foundation is a nonprofit organization that provides patients with practical information and coping strategies to minimize the effects of Sjögren's syndrome. The Web site offers support for people with Sjögren's syndrome and their families. The Foundation promotes public awareness, provides education for health professionals, and supports ongoing research.

The American Liver Foundation
75 Maiden Lane, Suite 603
New York, NY 10038
Ph: 800–GO–Liver (465–4837) (toll-free)
Ph: 888–4HEP–USA (443–7872) (toll-free)
Ph: 212–668–1000
www.liverfoundation.org

This nonprofit organization is dedicated to the prevention of liver diseases by providing education, research information, and advocacy on behalf of those at risk of or affected by liver disease.

American Academy of Allergy, Asthma & Immunology
611 East Wells Street
Milwaukee, WI 53202
Ph: 414–272–6071
www.aaaai.org

This Web site offers the latest information in the area of allergy, asthma, and immunology and a directory of specialists.

American Association for Chronic Fatigue Syndrome
27 N. Wacker Drive, Suite 416
Chicago, IL 60606
Ph: 847–258–7248 (voice mail)
www.aacfs.org

This nonprofit organization is comprised of research scientists and healthcare professionals whose interest is in promoting educational material and exchanging ideas about chronic fatigue syndrome, (CFS) and Fibromyalgia (FM) research, and patient care. It offers information through current periodic reviews of new clinical research and treatment ideas for the benefit of chronic fatigue syndrome and Fibromyalgia patients and others.

American Chronic Pain Association
PO Box 850
Rocklin, CA 95677
Ph: 800–533–3231
www.theacpa.org

This organization works to help people better manage their pain and live more satisfying, productive lives. The Web site offers information about pain management and stories from people with chronic pain, and how they have learned to live well in spite of their pain.

Neuroland
www.neuroland.com

This Web site offers a variety of information on conditions of the central nervous system and about clinical neurology.

Med Help International
6300 North Wickham Road
Suite 130, PMB #188
Melbourne, FL 32940
Ph: 321–259–7505
www.medhelp.org

This organization provides online medical information to patients and family members to help them make informed decisions on

*treatment Visitors to the Web site can ask questions of top medical
doctors from the best healthcare institutions around the world. In
addition, there is an online "Medical Community Forum" where you
can get medical advice and support from others with similar
experience or conditions.*

U.S. Government Web Sites

National Institute of Arthritis and Musculoskeletal and Skin
    Diseases
National Institutes of Health
1 AMS Circle
Bethesda, MD 20892–3675
Ph: 301–495–4484 or 877–22–NIAMS (toll-free)
TTY: 301–565–2966
www.niams.nih.gov

*National Institute of Arthritis and Musculoskeletal and Skin Diseases
is a government agency that serves the public, patients, and health
professionals by providing information, locating other information
sources, creating health information materials, and participating in a
national federal database on health information. This Web site offers a
variety of information related to rheumatologic conditions.*

U.S. National Library of Medicine-Medline Plus
www.nlm.nih.gov/medlineplus
*This Web site of the National Library of Medicine contains a large
amount of information on lupus and related disorders. It includes
general information, treatments, general health news, and more.*

Social Security Administration (Disability Information)
6401 Security Blvd.,
Baltimore, MD 21235–0001

1–800–772–1213

www.ssa.gov

This Web site provides information related to the organization and function of the Social Security Administration, of the Commissioner of Social Security, press releases, and how to contact the Social Security Administration's regional offices.

Social Security Administration (Employment Support Programs)
Office of Public Inquiries
Windsor Park Building
6401 Security Blvd.
Baltimore, MD 21235
Ph: 800–772–1213
TTY: 800–325–0778 (for deaf or hard of hearing)
www.ssa.gov/work

This Web site provides information on the programs, projects, and policies of the Social Security Administration related to employment support. This includes information about vocational rehabilitation service providers and organizations in every state that assist Social Security Administration disability beneficiaries with making choices about work by providing free advice and information on vocational rehabilitation. The site also includes information about Social Security Administration's Vocational Rehabilitation Payment Program, Employment and Vocational Rehabilitation Service Providers, and links to public rehabilitation agencies, employment services, and legal advice.

Food and Drug Administration
5600 Fishers Lane
Rockville, MD 20857
www.fda.gov

This agency regulates food, drugs, medical devices, and biologics, (vaccine, blood products, etc.), and assures its safety for the public use. This Web site provides information on the various agencies under the auspices of the Food and Drug Administration.

US Equal Employment Opportunity Commission
1801 L Street, NW
Washington, DC 20507
Ph: 1–800–669–4000 (voice)
TTD: 1–800–669–6820
Ph: 202–663–4900 (voice)
TDD: 202–663–4494
http://www.eeoc.gov/facts/ada18.html

This Web site provides an explanation of the Americans with Disabilities Act (ADA) rules that prohibit job discrimination ("Your Employment Rights as an Individual with a Disability: It is unlawful to discriminate in employment against a qualified individual with a disability."). This part of the law is enforced by the U.S. Equal Employment Opportunity Commission and state and local civil rights enforcement agencies that work with the commission. The Americans with Disabilities Act also prohibits discrimination against individuals with disabilities in state and local government services, public accommodations, transportation, and telecommunications.

Centers for Medicare & Medicaid Services
7500 Security Boulevard
Baltimore, MD 21244–1850
Medicaid Federal Information Clearinghouse
www.cms.hhs.gov/medicaid/default.asp
Medicare Federal Information Clearinghouse

www.medicare.gov/contacts/home.asp

Medicaid and Medicare are programs that pay for medical assistance for qualified individuals and families with low incomes and limited resources. These Web sites will provide you with the information required for qualification to the programs and other resources.

National Women's Health Information Center
Ph: 800–994–WOMAN (800–994–9662) (toll-free)
TTY: 888–220–5446

www.4woman.gov

This Web site and toll-free call center were created to provide free, reliable health information for women everywhere. It contains a database that serves as a great resource of information related to women, including such topics as heart disease, disabilities, and pregnancy.

Office on Women's Health
Department of Health and Human Services
200 Independence Avenue SW, Room 730B
Washington, DC 20201
Ph: 202–690–7650

www.4woman.gov/owh/index.htm

The Office on Women's Health (OWH) of the Department of Health and Human Services is the government office that addresses women's health issues and healthcare services. It examines how inequities in research can place the health of women at risk. Office on Women's Health coordinates women's efforts to eliminate disparities in healthcare and supports culturally sensitive educational programs to encourage women to take personal responsibility for their own health and wellness.

Miscellaneous Resources

Sun Protective Clothing Ltd.
598 Norris Court
Kingston, Ontario K7P 2R9 Canada
Ph: 613–384–3230 or 800–353–8778 (toll-free)
www.sunprotectiveclothing.com

This Web site offers products from a company that specializes in clothing that provides protection from the sun.

Sun Clothing, Etc.
907 Charles Street
Fredericksburg, VA 22401
Ph: 540–373–7175 or 866–713–9352 (toll-free)
www.sunclothingetc.com

This is another company that sells sun protection clothing.

Masque Rays, Inc.
3525 Del Mar Heights Road
San Diego, CA 92130
Ph: 858–756–6882 or 877–SunSuit (877–786–7848) (toll-free)
www.sunproof.com

This company offers sun protection clothing for children and adults.

Sun Precautions
2815 Wetmore Avenue
Everett, WA 98201
Ph: 425–303–8585 or 800–882–7860 (toll-free)
www.sunprecautions.com

This is a large company that sells sun protection clothing for the entire family.

The Comfort Store
7719 Graphics Way, Suite A
Lewis Center, OH 43035
Ph: 740–549–3900 or 888–867–2225 (toll-free)
www.sitincomfort.com

This company sells a selection of accessories for your comfort and protection.

Healthy Legs
Ph: 888–495–0105 (toll-free)
www.healthylegs.com

This company sells support hose and stockings for women and men of all ages.

My Foot Shop
Ph: 888–859–8901 (toll-free)
www.myfootshop.com

This company sells a large selection of products to take care of your feet.

DermaDoctor.com
Ph: 877–DERMADR (877–337–6237) (toll-free)
www.dermadoctor.com

This company has a large selection of sunblock and other skin products.

Skin Therapy Letter
http://www.skintherapyletter.com/

This Web site provides a detailed explanation on the importance of sunscreens and the factors that may affect the products that you may be using. It helps customers select the sunscreen best suited to their condition.

DermIS
http://dermis.net

This Web site offers a variety of information on skin conditions, as well as the risk factors, treatments, and prevention of skin diseases.

DoctorDirectory.com
www.doctordirectory.com

This Web site provides a directory to help locate physicians in any specialty in any region of the nation.

Doctor-Patient Communication Tips

Quackwatch
www.quackwatch.org/02ConsumerProtection/commtips.html

This Web site offers ideas on how the patient can maintain clear, effective communication with his/her physician or healthcare team.

American Medical Association Doctors Finder
http://dbapps.ama-assn.org/aps/amahg.htm

This Web site helps patients locate physicians by their specialty.

Discoveryhealth.com
http://health.discovery.com/encyclopedias/medical/medical.html

This Web site offers information about the various medical tests that physicians order as part of patient care.

Global RPH

www.globalrph.com/labinter.htm

This Web site provides the normal values of the blood tests frequently performed by physicians.

MedicineNet.com

www.medicinenet.com

This Web site provides medical information related to diagnoses, symptoms, laboratories, treatments, and procedures.

Health Gazette

www.tfn.net/HealthGazette/labwork2.html

This Web site provides information about the meaning or interpretation of the laboratory results.

MedBioWorld

www.medbioworld.com/med/journals/med-bio.html

This Web site offers the largest medical and bioscience information resource on the Internet, providing access to more than 25,000 active links to medical and bioscience journals, associations, databases, and other medical resources.

Clinical Trials and Research

Stem Cell Information

http://stemcells.nih.gov

This Web site offers information about stem cell treatments, clinical trials, and ongoing research.

ClinicalTrials.gov
http://clinicaltrials.gov

This Web site contains approximately 10,000 clinical studies sponsored by the National Institutes of Health, other federal agencies, and private industry. The studies are conducted in all fifty states and in more than ninety countries. The information is frequently updated. An individual wishing to participate in any of these trials will find information on the trial's purpose, who may participate, locations, and phone numbers to call for more details.

National Institute of Arthritis and Musculoskeletal and Skin
    Diseases
National Institutes of Health
www.niams.nih.gov/hi/registry/registry.htm

This Web site provides contact information for a variety of clinical studies in which you can participate on lupus and related conditions. Some of the studies are alopecia areata, ankylosing spondylitis, antiphospholipid syndrome, epidermolysis bullosa, fibromyalgia, ichthyosis, juvenile dermatomyositis, juvenile rheumatoid arthritis, muscular dystrophy, neonatal lupus, rheumatoid arthritis, and scleroderma.

Hamline University
1536 Hewitt Avenue
Saint Paul, MN 55104
Ph: 651–523–2800
www.hamline.edu/lupus

This Web site provides information about lupus and other research studies in which one can participate.

Lupus Study and Repository
Ph: 888–OK-LUPU (888–655–8787)
http://lupus.omrf.ouhsc.edu

Lupus Foundation of Minnesota
Ph: 800–51–LUPUS (800–515–8787)
*The Division of Rheumatology at the University of Minnesota is
conducting genetic research on lupus. It is looking for individuals
with lupus or families with two or more family members with lupus
to participate in its lupus genetic studies.*

Antiphospholipid Syndrome National Registry
National Institutes of Health
www.niams.nih.gov/ne/press/2001/04_19.htm
Ph: 301–496–8190

*This Web page includes a registry designed to benefit patients with
antiphospholipid syndrome. Anyone wanting to participate in this
research will find the contact information to apply to enter in the
study, and general information about antiphospholipid syndrome.*

Pharmaceutical Company Sites

La Jolla Pharmaceutical Company
6455 Nancy Ridge Drive
San Diego, CA 92121–2249
Ph: 858–452–6600
www.ljpc.com

*This Web site provides information on La Jolla's therapies for
antibody-mediated autoimmune diseases afflicting several million
people in the United States and Europe. The company is developing a*

treatment for patients with lupus, kidney disease, antibody-mediated thrombosis (a condition in which patients suffer from recurrent stroke, deep vein thrombosis, and other thrombotic events), and others. There is also information about La Jolla's clinical trials with these new drugs.

Partnership for Prescription Assistance
www.pparx.org

This Web site will help you find patient-assistance programs for prescription medicines for which you may qualify. On this interactive Web site, Pharmaceutical Research and Manufacturers of America and forty-eight member pharmaceutical companies offer an online directory of prescription drug patient-assistance programs that are supported by pharmaceutical companies. Some of the patient-assistance programs for specific prescribed medications in rheumatology are presented in the following table. (Note: Neither the author nor the publisher of this book endorse any of the products or manufacturers listed below.)

TABLE

Drug Name (Brand Name)	Manufacturer	Program Contact Information
Acetaminophen (Tylenol®)	Ortho McNeil	Ortho-McNeil Patient Assistance Program P.O. Box 938 Somerville, NJ 08876 800-797-7737

Drug Name (Brand Name)	Manufacturer	Program Contact Information
Adalimumab (Humira®)	Abbott Immunology	866-4-HUMIRA
Alendronate (Fosamax®)	Merck	The Merck Patient Assistance Program 800-994-2111 (Healthcare professionals only)
Celecoxib (Celebrex®)	Pfizer Inc	Connection to Care 800-707-8990 www.pfizer.com Pfizer for Living Share Card Program 800-717-6005 www.pfizerforliving.com Sharing the Care 800-984-1500 www.pfizer.com
Cyclosporine (Neoral®)	Novartis	Novartis Pharmaceuticals Patient Assistance Program P.O. Box 8609 Somerville, NJ 08876 800-277-2254
Etanercept (Enbrel®)	Amgen and Wyeth	Pharmaceuticals ENcourage Foundation™ 888-4ENBREL
Etidronate (Didronel®)	Procter & Gamble	Procter & Gamble Pharmaceuticals C/O Express Scripts, P.O. Box 6553 St. Louis, MO 63166-6553 800-830-9049

continued on the next page

Table, continued

Drug Name (Brand Name)	Manufacturer	Program Contact Information
Gamimune®	Bayer Corporation	Pharmaceutical Division Bayer Indigent Program P.O. Box 29209 Phoenix, AZ 85038-9209 800-998-9180 or 800-468-0894, Ext. 2765
Infliximab (Remicade®)	Centocor, US	REMICADE® PATIENT ASSISTANCE PROGRAM P.O. Box 221709 Charlotte, NC 28222-1709 866-489-5957 866-489-5958 (Fax)
Lansoprazole (Prevacid®)	TAP Pharmaceuticals, Inc	800-830-1015
Leflunomide (Arava®)	Aventis Pharmaceuticals	Aventis Pharmaceuticals Patient Assistance Program P.O. Box 759 Somerville, NJ 08876 800-221-4025
Meloxicam (Mobic®)	Boehringer Ingelheim Pharmaceuticals, Inc.	Boehringer Ingelheim Cares Foundation, Inc. c/o ESI/SDS P.O. Box 66555 St. Louis, MO 63166-6773 800-556-8317
Mycophenolate Mofetil (CellCept®)	Roche	Roche Medical Needs Program Roche Laboratories, Inc 340 Kingsland Street Nutley, NJ 07110 800-285-4484

Drug Name (Brand Name)	Manufacturer	Program Contact Information
Nabumetone (Relafen®)	GlaxoSmithKline	SmithKline Beecham Foundation Access to Care c/o Express Scrits/SDS P.O. Box 2564 Maryland Heights, MO 63043-8564 800-546-0420 800-729-4544 (Fax)
Naproxen (Naprosyn®)	Roche	Roche Medical Needs Program Roche Laboratories, Inc 340 Kingsland Street Nutley, NJ 07110 800-285-4484
Nitrofurantoin (Macrodantin®, Macrobid®)	Procter & Gamble	Procter & Gamble Pharmaceuticals C/O Express Scripts P.O. Box 6553 St. Louis, MO 63166-6553 800-830-9049
Omeprazole (Prilosec®)	AstraZeneca	Patient Assistance Program AstraZeneca Foundation P.O. Box 15197 Wilmington, DE 19850-5197 800-424-3727
Paroxetine (Paxil®)	GlaxoSmithKline	SmithKline Beecham Foundation Access to Care c/o Express Scrits/SDS P.O. Box 2564 Maryland Heights, MO 63043-8564 1-800-546-0420 1-800-729-4544 (Fax)
Raloxifene (Evista®)	Eli Lilly and Company	www.lillyanswers.com 877-795-4559

continued on the next page

Table, continued

Drug Name (Brand Name)	Manufacturer	Program Contact Information
Risedronate (Actonel®)	Procter & Gamble	Procter & Gamble Pharmaceuticals P.O. Box 6553 St. Louis, MO 63166–6553 800–830–9049
Rituximab (Rituxan®)	Genentech, Inc.	Genentech Access to Care Foundation 1 DNA Way South San Francisco, CA 94080–4990 800–530–3083 650–225–1366 (Fax)
Rofecoxib (Vioxx®)	Merck	The Merck Patient Assistance Program 800–994–2111 (Healthcare professionals only)
Teriparatide (Forteo®)	Eli Lilly and Company	*www.lillyanswers.com* 877–795–4559
Tramadol (Ultram®, Ultracet®)	Ortho McNeil	Ortho-McNeil Patient Assistance Program P.O. Box 938 Somerville, NJ 08876 800–797–7737
Valdecoxib (Bextra®)	Pfizer Inc	Connection to Care 800–707–8990 www.pfizer.com Pfizer for Living Share Card Program 800–717–6005 *www.pfizerforliving.com* Sharing the Care 800–984–1500 *www.pfizer.com*

International Lupus Organizations

This section is of value to those patients who may need to move to other countries. These organizations are located in various parts of the world and will help you stay in contact with other lupus groups and participate in lupus activities while living outside of the United States.

International League of Associations for Rheumatology
www.ilar.org

International League of Associations for Rheumatology is the global umbrella organization devoted to the treatment and prevention of rheumatic diseases worldwide. It pursues this activity mainly through its relationship with the Regional Leagues (PANLAR, EULAR, APLAR, and AFLAR). One of its main activities is the promotion of education of medical personnel, other health professionals, and the public. Contact information will depend on the regional area: PANLAR, EULAR, APLAR, or AFLAR.

Lupus Around the World
www.mtio.com/lupus

This Web site provides the information needed to cope with chronic illness: up-to-date information, immediate support by others in similar situations, and links to every other lupus-related site on the Web.

Lupus Canada
18 Crown Steel DR Suite 209
Markham ON L3R 9X8 Canada
Ph: 905–513–0004 or 800–661–1468 (toll-free in Canada)
www.lupuscanada.org

This Web site is a source of information about lupus organizations in Canada and information about lupus in general.

European Lupus Erythematosus Federation
www.elef.rheumanet.org
E-mail: *elef@rheumanet.org*

This is a group of European lupus organizations representing the lupus patients of fifteen countries. They offer information about lupus and activities in their respective areas.

Lupus UK
www.lupusuk.com

Lupus UK provides information about lupus in the United Kingdom on its Web site, including the latest dates for national and international meetings.

St. Thomas' Lupus Trust
Rayne Institute
St. Thomas' Hospital
London SE1 7EH United Kingdom
Ph: 020 7922 8197
www.lupus.org.uk

The Web site of St. Thomas' Hospital, in the center of London, offers information about lupus and the clinic, which follows approximately 2,500 lupus patients.

Association Française du Lupus et autres Collagenoses (A.F.L.)
(French Association of Lupus and Systemic Rheumatic Disease)
25 Rue des Charmettes
F 69100 Villeurbanne France
Ph: +33–04–72 74 10 86
www.elef.rheumanet.org/register/r-fra.htm

This Web site provides information in English and French for lupus patients who wish to participate in group activities.

Liga voor Chronische Inflammatoire Bindweefselziekten
    (CIBliga)
(Belgian league for chronic inflammation: lupus,
Sjögren's syndrome, scleroderma, poly- or dermatomyositis,
vasculitis and MCTD)
Bijendries 20, 3530 Houthalen Belgium
Ph/fax: (011) 72 79 52
www.CIBliga.com

This Web site provides information on lupus, links, resources, and support in Belgium.

SLE ryhma (Finnish lupus group)
Iso Roobertinkatu 20–22 A
FIN 00120 Helsinki Finland
Ph: +358–9– 4761 5601
www.elef.rheumanet.org/register/r-fin.htm

This Web site provides contact information about the lupus group in Finland.

Lupus Erythematodes Selbsthilfegemeinschaft e.V. (Germany
    Lupus Lupus Erythematodes Selbsthilfegemeinschaft e.V.
    (German lupus association)
Döppersberg 20
42103 Wuppertal Germany
Ph: +49–202–496 87 97
www.elef.rheumanet.org/register/r-ger.htm

This Web site gives you the information to contact the lupus group in Germany.

KJARNINN, ahugahopur um Lupus (Iceland rheumatism league)
Armuli 5
108 Reykjavik Iceland
Ph: +354–553–07 60
www.elef.rheumanet.org/register/r–ice.htm

This Web site provides contact information about the lupus group in Iceland.

Gruppo Italiano per la lotta contro il lupus eritematoso sistemico (Italian lupus group)
www.lupus–italy.org
Gruppo Italiano per la Lotta contro il
Lupus Eritematoso Sistemico ONLUS
Via Arbotori, 14 - 29100 Piacenza – I Italy
Ph/Fax: +39 0523 753643

This organization provides you with lupus information, activities, and resources of the lupus group in Italy.

Nationale Vereniging LE Patienten (Dutch national society of lupus patients)
Bisonspoor 3004
NL-3605 LV Maarssen Netherlands
Ph: +31–346–55 24 01
www.elef.rheumanet.org/register/r–net.htm

This Web site provides information in English and Dutch about the lupus group in the Netherlands.

Lupus Foreningen i NRF (Norwegian lupus foundation within
 NRF)
Aassvangveien 6B
N-9360 Bardu Norway
Ph.: +47–77 18 19 25
www.elef.rheumanet.org/register/r-nor.htm

*This Web site provides information in English and Norweigan
about the lupus group in Norway.*

Federación Española de Lupus (Spanish lupus federation)
C/ Lagunillas, 25
Locales 3 y 4
Málaga 29012 Spain
Ph.: +34–95–226 65 04 or +34–95 225 08 26
www.elef.rheumanet.org/register/r-spa.htm

*This Web site offers information in English and Spanish about the
lupus group in Spain.*

SLE/Sjögrenrådet - Rheumatikerförbundet (Swedish lupus and
 Sjögren group)
Sandbackavägen 32L
903 46 Umeå Sweden
Ph: +46–90–13 00 65 or 46–739–1646 83
www.elef.rheumanet.org/register/r-swe.htm

*This Web site offers information in English and Swedish about the
lupus group in Sweden.*

Irgun Ha-lupus Lelsrael (Israeli lupus association)
P.O. Box 14103
Tel Aviv Israel

Ph: +972–4–854 28 89

www.elef.rheumanet.org/register/r–isr.htm

This Web site provides contact information in English and in Hebrew about the lupus group in Israel.

Associação de Doentes com Lupus (Portuguese association of
    patients with lupus)
Praça Francisco
Sá Carneiro No. 11, 2./ Esq.
1000–160 Lisboa Portugal
Ph: +351–1–846 44 83

www.elef.rheumanet.org/register/r–por.htm

This Web site offers you information in English and Portuguese about the lupus group in Portugal.

Lupus Australia, Qld Inc.
P.O. Box 974
Kenmore Q 4069 Australia
Ph: (07) 38789553

www.lupus.com.au

This Web site offers information about the lupus groups and other resources in Australia.

SELECTED REFERENCES

In this section readers are offered the opportunity to look for other sources of information. These are published manuscripts related to different aspects of lupus, such as the clinical manifestations, the environmental influences, and research findings. Within each publication you will find another set of references that were used by each author. The manuscripts are listed in alphabetical order by author, followed by the title of the article, the journal in which you can find it, the volume number, the page numbers, and the year of publication. You can find a copy of many of these manuscripts on the Web, at your local library, or by writing directly to the authors.

Alarcón GS, Friedman AW, Straaton KV, Moulds JM, Lisse J, Bastian HM, McGwin GJR, Bartolucci AA, Roseman JM, Reville JD. Systemic lupus erythematosus in three ethnic groups: III A comparison of characteristics early in the natural history of the LUMINA cohort. *Lupus.* 8: 197–209; 1999.

Arkachaisri T, Lehman TJA. Systemic lupus erythematosus and related disorders of childhood. *Current Opinion in Rheumatology.* 11: 384–392; 1999.

Arnal C, Piette JC, Leone J, Taillan B, Hachulla E, Roudot-Thoraval F, Papo T, Schaeffer A, Bierling P, Godeau B. Treatment of severe immune thrombocytopenia associated with systemic lupus erythematosus. *Journal of Rheumatology.* 29: 75–83; 2002.

Arnett FC, Hamilton RG, Roebber M, Harley JB, Reichlin M. Increased frequencies of Sm and nRNP autoantibodies in American blacks compared to whites with systemic lupus erythematosus. *Journal of Rheumatology.* 15: 1773–1776; 1988.

Arnett FC, Shulman LE. Studies in familial systemic lupus erythematosus. *Medicine.* 55: 13–321; 1976.

Atkinson RA, Appenzeller O. Headache in small vessel disease of the brain: A study of patterns with systemic lupus erythematosus. *Headache.* 5: 198–201; 1975.

Austin HA 3d, Klippel JH, Balow JE, et al. Therapy of lupus
    nephritis: controlled trial of prednisone and cytotoxic drugs.
    New England Journal of Medicine. 314: 614–619; 1986.

Backos M, Rai R, Baxter N, Chilcott IT, Cohen H, Regan L.
    Pregnancy complications in woman with recurrent
    miscarriage associated with antiphospholipid antibodies
    treated with low dose aspirin and heparin. *British Journal of
    Obstetrics and Gynaecology.* 106: 102–107; 1999.

Baden HP, Pearlman C. The effects of ultraviolet light on
    protein and nucleic acid synthesis in the epidermis. *Journal
    of Dermatology.* 43: 71–75; 1964.

Bakir AA, Levy PS, Dunea G. The prognosis of lupus nephritis
    in African-Americans: A retrospective analysis. *American
    Journal of Kidney Diseases.* 24: 159–171; 1994.

Ballou SP, Khan MA, Kushner I. Clinical features of systemic
    lupus erythematosus: Differences related to race and age of
    onset. *Arthritis & Rheumatism.* 25: 55–61; 1982.

Beer KR, Lorincz AL, Medenica MM, Albertini J, Baron J,
    Drinkard L, Swartz T. Insecticide-induced lupus
    erythematosus. *International Journal of Dermatology.* 33:
    860–862; 1994.

Berden JHM. Lupus Nephritis. *Kidney International.* 52:
    538–558; 1997.

Bigazzi PE. Autoimmunity induced by chemicals. *Clinical
    Toxicology.* 26: 125–156; 1988.

Block SR, Winfield JB, Lockshin MD, D'Angelo WA,
    Christian CL. Studies of twins with systemic lupus. A
    review of the literature and presentation of 12 additional
    sets. *American Journal of Medicine.* 59: 533–552; 1975.

Brewster JA, Shaw NJ, Farquharson RG. Neonatal and pediatric outcome of infants born to mothers with antiphospholipid syndrome. *Journal of Perinatal Medicine.* 27: 183–187; 1999.

Buckman KJ, Moore SK, Ebbin M, Cox MB, Dubois FL. Familial systemic lupus erythematosus. *Archive of Internal Medicine.* 138: 1674–1676; 1978.

Chaplin H, Avioli LV. Autoimmune hemolytic anemia. *Archive of Internal Medicine.* 137: 346–352; 1977.

Clark WF, Kortas C, Heidenheim AP, Garland J, Spanner E, Parbtani A. Flaxseed in lupus nephritis: A two year placebo controlled crossover study. *Journal of the American College of Nutrition.* 20: 143–148; 2001.

Cooper GS, Dooley MA, Treadwell EL, St. Clair EW, Parks CG, Gilkeson GS. Hormonal, environmental, and infectious risk factors for developing systemic lupus erythematosus. *Arthritis & Rheumatism.* 41(10): 1714–1724; 1998.

Cooper GS, Dooley MA, Treadwell EL, St. Clair EW, Parks CG, Gilkeson GS. Smoking and use of hair treatment in relation to risk of developing systemic lupus erythematosus. *Journal of Rheumatology.* 28: 2653–2656; 2001.

Delbarre F, Pompidou A, Hahan A, Brouihlet H, LeGo A, Amor B. Study of lymphocytes during systemic lupus erythematosus. *Pathology and Biology.* 19: 379–385; 1971.

Deuel T, Gardner F, Peck WA. Thrombotic thrombocytopenia purpura. *Archive of Internal Medicine.* 140: 93–95; 1980.

Dimant J, Ginzler EM, Schlesinger M, Diamond HS, Kaplan D. Systemic lupus erythematosus in the older age group: computer analysis. *Journal of the American Geriatric Society.* 27: 58–61; 1979.

Donadio JV, Glassock RJ. Immunosuppressive drug therapy in
    lupus nephritis. *American Journal of Kidney Disease* 21:
    239–250; 1993.

Dooley MA, Hogan SL. Environmental epidemiology and risk
    factors for autoimmune disease. *Current Opinion of
    Rheumatology.* 15: 99–103; 2003.

Dubois EL. Acquired hemolytic anemia as presenting syndrome
    of lupus erythematosus disseminatus. *American Journal of
    Medicine.* 22: 197–204; 1952.

Elkon KB, Bonfa E, Weisshbach H, et al. Neuropsychiatric
    manifestations of systemic lupus erythematosus. *British
    Journal of Rheumatology* 291: 6; 1993.

Ellis SG, Verity MA. Central nervous system involvement in
    systemic lupus erythematosus: A review of neuropathologic
    findings in 57 cases, 1955–1977. *Seminars of Arthritis &
    Rheumatism.* 8: 212–221; 1979.

Esplin S. Management of antiphospholipid syndrome during
    pregnancy. *Clinical Obstetrics and Gynecology.* 44: 20–28;
    2001.

Eyanson S, Passo MH, Aldo-Benson MA, Benson MD.
    Methylprednisolone pulse therapy for nonrenal lupus
    erythematosus. *Annals of Rheumatic Diseases.* 39: 377–380;
    1980.

Fessel WJ. Epidemiology of systemic lupus erythematosus.
    Rheumatic Clinics of North America. 14: 15–23; 1988.

Fox DA, McCune WJ. Immunosuppressive drug therapy of
    systemic lupus erythematosus. *Rheumatic Disease Clinics of
    North America.* 20: 265; 1994.

Furner BB. Treatment of subacute cutaneous lupus
    erythematosus. *International Journal of Dermatology.* 29: 542;
    1990.

Gattorno M, Molinari AC, Buoncompagni A, Acquila M, Amato S, Picco P. Recurrent antiphospholipid-related deep vein thrombosis as presenting manifestation of systemic lupus erythematosus. *European Journal of Pediatrics*. 159: 211–214; 2000.

Gibson T, Myers AR. Nervous system involvement in systemic lupus erythematosus. *Annals of Rheumatic Diseases*. 35: 398–406; 1976.

Gillian JN, Sontheimer RD. Skin manifestations of SLE. *Clinics of Rheumatology Disease*. 6: 207; 1982.

Gruenberg JC, VanSlyck EJ, Abraham JP. Splenectomy in systemic lupus erythematosus. *American Surgery*. 52: 366–370; 1986.

Harley JB, Moser KL, Gaffney PM, Behrens TW. The genetics of human systemic lupus erythematosus. *Current Opinion of Immunology*. 10: 690–696; 1998.

Harley JB, Sheldon P, Neas B, Murphy S, Wallace DJ, Scofield RH, Shaver TS, Moser KL. Systemic lupus erythematosus: considerations for a genetic approach. *Journal of Investigational Dermatology*. 103: 144S-149S; 1994.

Harvey AM, Shulman LE, Tumulty PA, Conley CL, Schoenrich EH. Systemic lupus erythemaotsus: Review of the literature and clinical analysis of 138 cases. *Medicine*. (Baltimore) 33: 291–437; 1954.

Hess EV, Farhey Y. Etiology, environmental relationship, epidemiology, and genetics of systemic lupus erythematosus. *Current Opinion of Rheumatology*. 7: 371–375; 1995.

Hirose W, Fukuya H, Anzai T, Kawagoe M, Kawai T, Watanabe K. Myelofibrosis and systemic lupus erythematosus. *Journal of Rheumatology*. 20: 2164–2166; 1993.

Hochberg MC. Updating the American College of
Rheumatology Criteria for systemic lupus erythematosus.
Arthritis & Rheumatism. 41: 751; 1998.

Hochberg MC, Boyd RE, Ahream JM, Arnett FC, Bias WB,
Proost TT, Stevens MB. Systemic lupus erythematosus: a
review of clinico-laboratory features and immunogenetic
markers in 150 patients with emphasis on demographic
subsets. *Medicine.* 64: 285–295; 1985.

Hutchinson GA, Nehall JE, Simeon DT. Psychiatric disorders
in systemic lupus erythematosus. *West Indian Medical
Journal.* 45: 48; 1996.

Iverson GL, Anderson KW. The etiology of psychiatric
symptoms in patients with systemic lupus erythematosus.
Scandinavian Journal of Rheumatology. 23: 277; 1994.

James JA, Harley JB, Scofield RH. Role of viruses in systemic
lupus erythematosus and Sjögren's syndrome. *Current
Opinion of Rheumatology.* 13: 370–376; 2001.

James JA, Kaufman KM, Farris AD, Taylor-Albert E, Lechman
TJA, Harley JB. An increased prevalence of Epstein-Barr
virus infection in young patients suggests a possible etiology
for systemic lupus erythematosus. *Journal of Clinical
Investigation.* 100: 3019–3026; 1997.

Kiss E, Gal I, Simkovics E, Kiss A, Banyai A, Szakall S,
Szegedi G. Myelofibrosis in systemic lupus erythematosus.
Leukemia Lymphoma. 39: 661–665; 2000.

Laversuch CJ, Collins DA, Charles PJ, Bourke BE.
Sulphasalazine-induced autoimmune abnormalities in
patients with rheumatic diseases. *British Journal of
Rheumatology* 34: 435–439; 1995.

Lee, Silver RM. Recurrent pregnancy loss: Summary and clinical recommendations. *Seminars of Reproductive Medicine.* 18: 433–440; 2000.

Lee T, Scheven EV, Sandborg C. Systemic lupus erythematosus and antiphospholipid syndrome in children and adolescents. *Current Opinion of Rheumatology.* 13: 415–421; 2001.

Love LA. New environmental agents associated with lupus-like disorders. *Lupus.* 3: 367–471; 1994.

Manson JJ, Isenberg DA. The pathogenesis of systemic lupus erythematosus. *The Journal of Medicine.* 61: 343–346; 2003.

McAlindon T, Giannotta L, Taub N, D'Cruz D, Hughes G. Environmental factors predicting nephritis in systemic lupus erythematosus. *Annals of Rheumatic Diseases.* 52: 720–724: 1993.

McCune WJ, Golbus J, Zeldes W, et al: Clinical and immunologic effects of monthly administration of intravenous cyclophosphamide in severe systemic lupus erythematosus. *New England Journal of Medicine.* 318: 1423–1431; 1988.

McNicholl JM, Glynn D, Mongey AB, Hutchinson M, Bresnihan B. A prospective study of neurophysiologic, neurologic and immunologic abnormalities in systemic lupus erythematosus. *Journal of Rheumatology.* 21: 1061–1066; 1994.

Miller MH, Urowitz MB, Gladman DD. The significance of thrombocytopenia in systemic lupus erythematosus. *Arthritis & Rheumatism.* 26: 1181–1186; 1983.

Mirzayan MJ, Schmidt RE, Witte T. Prognostic parameters for flare in systemic lupus erythematosus. *Rheumatology.* 39: 1316–1319; 2000.

Moake JK. Thrombotic thrombocytopenic purpura today. *Hospital Practice.* 15: 53–59; 1999.

Molina JF, Molina J, Garcia C, Gharavi AE, Wilson WA, Espinoza LR. Ethnic differences in the clinical expression of systemic lupus erythematosus. *Lupus.* 6: 63–67; 1997.

Morgan M, Downs K, Chesterman CN, Biggs JC. Clinical analysis of 125 patients with the lupus anticoagulant. *Australia, New Zealand Journal of Medicine.* 23: 151; 1993.

Morteo OG, Franklin EC, McEwen C, Python J, Tanner M. Studies of relatives of patients with systemic lupus erythematosus. *Arthritis & Rheumatism.* 4: 356–361; 1961.

Moss KE, Isenberg DA. Comparison of renal disease severity and outcome in patients with primary antiphospholipid syndrome, antiphospholipid syndrome secondary to systemic lupus erythematosus and SLE alone. *Rheumatology.* 40: 863–867; 2001.

Myones BL, McCurdy D. The antiphospholipid syndrome: immunologic and clinical aspects. Clinical spectrum and treatment. *Journal of Rheumatology.* 27: 20–28; 2000.

O'Connor JF, Musher DM. Central nervous system involvement in systemic lupus erythematosus. *Archive of Neurology.* 14: 157–164; 1966.

Petri M. The effect of race on incidence and clinical course in systemic lupus erythematosus: The Hopkins Lupus Cohort. *Journal of the American Medicine Women's Association.* 53: 9–12; 1998.

Pollak VE, Pirani CL, Schwartz FD. The natural history of the renal manifestations of systemic lupus erythematosus. *Journal of Laboratory and Clinical Medicine.* 63: 537; 1964.

Quintero AI, Bacino D, Kelly J, Aberle T, Harley JB. Familial systemic lupus erythematosus: A comparison of clinical and antibodies presentations in three ethnic groups. *Cellular and Molecular Biology.* 47: 1223–1227; 2001.

Quintero AI, Kelly JA, Kilpatrick J, James JA, Harley JB. The genetics of Systemic Lupus Erythematosus Stratified by Renal Disease: Linkage at 10q22.3 (SLEN1), 2q34–35 (SLEN2) and 11p15.6 (SLEN3). *Genes & Immunity.* 3 Supplement 1: S57–62; 2002.

Quintero AI, Miller V. Neurologic symptoms in children with Systemic Lupus Erythematosus. *Journal of Child Neurology.* 15: 803–807; 2000.

Rahman P, Gladman DD, Urowitz MB. Smoking interferes with efficacy of antimalarial therapy in cutaneous lupus. *Journal of Rheumatology.* 25: 1716–1719; 1998.

Rahman P, Urowitz MB, Gladman DD, Bruce IN, Genest J Jr. Contribution of traditional risk factors to coronary disease in patients with systemic lupus erythematosus. *Journal of Rheumatology.* 26: 2363–2368; 1999.

Reichlin M, Harley JB, Lockshin MD. Serologic studies of monozygotic twins with systemic lupus erythematosus. *Arthritis & Rheumatism.* 35: 457–464; 1992.

Reidenberg MM, Drayer DE, Lorenzo B, Strom BL, West SL, Snyder ES, Freundlich B, Stolley PD. Acetylation phenotypes and environmental chemical exposure of people with idiopathic systemic lupus erythematosus. *Arthritis & Rheumatism.* 36: 971–973; 1993.

Reveille JD, Bartolucci A, Alarcón GS. Prognosis in systemic lupus erythematosus. *Arthritis & Rheumatism.* 33: 37–48; 1990.

Ridolfi RL, Bell WR. Thrombotic thrombocytopenic purpura: report of 25 cases and review of the literature. *Medicine.* 60: 413–428; 1981.

Rihner M, Mcgrath H. Fluorescent light photosensitivity in patients with systemic lupus erythematosus. *Arthritis & Rheumatism.* 35: 949–952; 1992.

Rivero SJ, Diaz-Jouanen E, Alarcon-Segovia D. Lymphopenia in systemic lupus erythematosus. Clinical, diagnostic, and prognostic significance. *Arthritis & Rheumatism.* 21: 295–305; 1978.

Roldan R, Roman J, Lopez D, Gonzalez J, Sanchez C, Martinez F. Treatment of hemolytic anemia and severe thrombocytopenia with high-dose methylprednisolone and intravenous immunoglobulins in SLE. *Scandinavian Journal of Rheumatology.* 23: 218–219; 1994.

Ruiz-Irastorza G, Khamashta MA, Castellino G, Hughes GRV. Systemic lupus erythematosus. *The Lancet.* 357: 1027–1032; 2001.

Sergent JS, Lockshin MD, Klempner MS, Lipsky BA. Central nervous system disease in systemic lupus erythematosus: Therapy and prognosis. *American Journal of Medicine.* 58: 644–654; 1975.

Singh K, Gaiha M, Shome DK, Gupta VK, Anuradha S. The association of antiphospholipid antibodies with ischaemic stroke and myocardial infarction in young and their correlation: A preliminary study. *JAPI.* 49: 527–529; 2001.

Sutej PG, Gear AJ, Morrison RCA, Tikly M, DeBeer M, Dos Santos L, Sher R. Photosensitivity and anti-Ro (SS-A) antibodies in black patients with systemic lupus erythematosus (SLE). *British Journal of Rheumatology.* 28: 321–324; 1989.

Tan EM, Cohen AS, Fries JF, Masi AT, McShane DJ, Rothfield NF, Schaller JG, Talal N, Winchester RJ. The 1982 revised criteria for the classification of systemic lupus erythematosus. *Arthritis & Rheumatism.* 25: 1271–1277; 1982.

Tripodi A, Mannuccio PM. Laboratory investigation of thrombophilia. *Clinical Chemistry.* 47: 1597–1606; 2001.

Vaiopoulos G, Sfikakis PP, Kapsimali V, Boki K, Panayiotidis P, Aessopos A, Tsokos GC, Kaklamanis P. The association of systemic lupus erythematosus and myasthenia gravis. *Postgraduate Medical Journal.* 70: 741–745; 1994.

Valesini G, Pittoni V. Treatment of thrombosis associated with immunological risk factors. *Annals of Medicine.* 32: 41–45; 2000.

Vial T, Nicolas B, Descotes J. Clinical immunotoxicity of pesticides. *Journal of Toxicology and Environmental Health.* 48: 215–229; 1996.

Vinatier D, Dufour P, Cosson M, Houpeau JL. Antiphospholipid syndrome and recurrent miscarriages. *European Journal of Obstetrics, Gynecology and Reproductive Biology.* 96: 37–50; 2001.

Wall BA, Weinblatt ME, Agudelo CA. Plasmapheresis in the treatment of resistant thrombocytopenia in systemic lupus erythematosus. *Southern Medical Journal.* 75: 1277–1278; 1982.

Wallace D. Management of lupus erythematosus: recent insights. *Current Opinion of Rheumatology.* 14: 212–219; 2002.

Walton AJE, Snaith ML, Locniskar M, Cumberland AG, Morrow WJW, Isenberg DA. Dietary fish oil and the severity of symptoms in patients with systemic lupus erythematosus. *Annals of Rheumatic Diseases.* 50: 463–466; 1991.

Ward MM, Pyan E, Studenski S. Mortality risks associated
    with specific clinical manifestations of systemic lupus
    erythematosus. *Archives of Internal Medicine.* 156:
    1337–1344; 1996.

Ward MM, Studenski S. Clinical prognostic factors in lupus
    nephritis. The importance of hypertension and smoking.
    Archives of Internal Medicine. 152: 2082–2088; 1992.

Watanabe T, Tsuchida T. Classification of lupus erythematosus
    based upon cutaneous manifestations. Dermatological,
    systemic and laboratory findings in 191 patients.
    Dermatology. 190: 277; 1995.

Wilson WA, Gharavi AE, Koike T, Lockshim MD, Branch
    DW, Piette JC, Brey R, Derksen R, Harris EN, Hughes
    GR, Triplett DA, Khamashta MA. International consensus
    statement on preliminary classification criteria for definite
    antiphospholipid syndrome. *Arthritis & Rheumatism.* 42:
    1309–1311; 1999.

Yamasaki K, Niho Y, Yanase T. Granulopoiesis in systemic lupus
    erythematosus. *Arthritis & Rheumatism.* 26: 516–521; 1983.

Yancy CL, Doughty RA, Athreya BH. Central nervous system
    involvement in childhood systemic lupus erythematosus.
    Arthritis & Rheumatism. 24: 1389–1395; 1981.